CORE CURRICULUM FOR MEDICAL QUALITY MANAGEMENT

AMERICAN COLLEGE OF MEDICAL QUALITY

JONES AND BARTLETT PUBLISHERS

Sudbury, Massachusetts

BOSTON   TORONTO   LONDON   SINGAPORE

World Headquarters
Jones and Bartlett Publishers
40 Tall Pine Drive
Sudbury, MA 01776
978-443-5000
info@jbpub.com
www.jbpub.com

Jones and Bartlett Publishers Canada
2406 Nikanna Road
Mississauga, ON L5C 2W6
CANADA

Jones and Bartlett Publishers International
Barb House, Barb Mews
London W6 7PA
UK

Library of Congress Cataloging-in-Publication Data

Core curriculum for medical quality management / American College of Medical Quality (ACMQ).
  p. ; cm.
 Includes bibliographical references and index.
 ISBN 0-7637-3061-0 (pbk.)
 1. Medical care-United States-Quality control-Outlines, syllabi, etc. 2. Total quality management-United States-Outlines, syllabi, etc.
 [DNLM: 1. Quality of Health Care-organization & administration. W 84 C797 2005] I. American College of Medical Quality.
 RA399.A3C667 2005
 362.1′068-dc22

                                                                                    2004029431

Production Credits
Executive Editor: Jack Bruggeman
Production Director: Amy Rose
Associate Production Editor: Renée Sekerak
Editorial Assistant: Kylah Goodfellow McNeill
Marketing Manager: Ed McKenna
Manufacturing and Inventory Coordinator: Amy Bacus
Composition and Art Creation: PD & PS
Printing and Binding: Malloy, Inc.
Cover Printing: Malloy, Inc.

Printed in the United States of America

09 08 07 06 05   10 9 8 7 6 5 4 3 2 1

CONTENTS

Chapter 1   Quality Management Principles and Practices   1
    ARTHUR L. PELBERG, MD, MPA

Chapter 2   Utilization Management   69

ERIC Z. SILFEN, MD, MHSA and

RALPH H ROSENBLUM, JR., DDS, MHA

Chapter 3   Organization Design and Management   95
JAMES T. ZIEGENFUSS, JR., PhD

Chapter 4   Economics, Finance, and Government in Medical Quality Management   123
DONALD FETTEROLF, MD, MBA and
JOSEPH L. BRAUN, MD, JD, MBA

Chapter 5   Medical Informatics and Information Systems:
The Information Infrastructure Needed to Support
Quality Measurement and Improvement   163
LOUIS H. DIAMOND, MB, CHB

Chapter 6 Legal and Ethical Issues in Medical
Quality Management   187
JOSEPH A. MISLOVE, JD, MBA and JEFFREY ZALE, MD, MPH

ABOUT THE AMERICAN COLLEGE MEDICAL QUALITY

For more than 30 years, the American College of Medical Quality (ACMQ) has been the physician-led organization dedicated to the measurement and improvement of quality in medicine.

With the mission of educating physicians and other health professionals in the evolving specialty of medical quality management, ACMQ is active in the American Medical Association House of Delegates with promoting quality issues to a wider physician audience.

The objectives of ACMQ's educational programs in medical quality management and clinical quality improvement are to develop and disseminate a core body of knowledge; provide a forum for health care professionals, government agencies, and other regulatory bodies; take a leadership role in creating, sustaining and applying a scientifically based infrastructure for the specialty; elevate the standards of medical schools and post-graduate education in quality management; and sponsor on-going research and evaluation.

George C. Martin, MD
ACMQ President, 2004–2005

ix

INTRODUCTION

Alex R. Rodriguez, MD
Chief Medical Officer
Magellan Health Services
Farmington, CT

During the modern era of medical quality management in the United States, there have been periodic efforts to compile the knowledge of the field into a compendium text, or "core curriculum." The first major effort, organized by John W. Williamson, MD, [1,2] in 1982, was ground-breaking because he and his colleagues recognized the critical need for a common language and beginning consensus about the concepts and methods that were rapidly emerging in the fields of medical utilization review and medical quality assurance. Indeed, before, and to some extent after, Dr. Williamson's first publication, a variety of texts focused on topical areas of health care quality management. [3–8] However, to date, only one previous book published under the auspices of medical specialty societies has attempted to collate the current understanding of medical quality management: *Health Care Quality Management for the 21st Century*,[9] edited by James Couch, MD, JD, for the American College of Medical Quality and American College of Physician Executives. Since the publication of this book in 1991, the knowledge base for medical quality has grown exponentially, as literally thousands of scholarly articles and books have been added to the canon of literature. Therefore, the American College of Medical Quality has determined that the health care provider and consumer communities now need and deserve a state-of-the-art update on the medical field that it leads.

In his seminal 1986 work *A Position Paper on the Future of ACURP*, Avedis Donabedian, MD, MPH, introduced a new medical specialty: clinical outcomes management. In this paper, Donabedian first articulated the core areas of knowledge that physicians in this field would require:[10]

1. Clinical competence: established training, experience, and certification in a clinical medical specialty, with a full understanding of relevant health ethics issues related to utilization and quality management.

2. The health care system and health institutions: requisite knowledge and experience in health care organizations' clinical services and administrative management.

xi

3. Performance review methods and systems: understanding of clinical performance assessment methods, including facility in medical criteria formulation, professional consensus development skills, disease and case-mix classifications, measurements of health status, and patient satisfaction.

4. Information systems: competence in hardware and software applications for data design, collection, and assessment.

5. Epidemiology and quantitative methods: understanding of epidemiologic measurement principles and biostatistics that would allow appropriate data analysis of health care quality, costs, and risk.

6. Organizational theory: facility in implementing quality management programs in complex organizations.

7. Adult education and organizational change: understanding of principles and methods for instructing patients and practitioners in ways that result in effective clinical decisions and desired health outcomes.

8. Health care law: basic competence in understanding aspects of the law that impact health systems, including risk management functions.

9. Institutional environmental health and safety: knowledge of issues that would affect risks to quality of care in organized settings where clinical services are provided.

10. Health economics: understanding of essential principles and methods that are relevant to health cost structures, processes, and outcomes.

While Dr. Donabedian was surmising what knowledge and skills would most likely be needed in educational programs, it now appears prophetic that he forecast a core curriculum for a specialty that, at the time, was in its most formative stages. He believed market and professional demands would soon result in a number of undergraduate and post-graduate medical quality training programs, and that these demands would fuel the supply of health services research, scholarly publications, and training programs for the new specialty. Given the profound challenges already facing a health care system burgeoning with demand and supply financial pressures, legal and regulatory activity, technological innovations, and public expectations for quality, affordability, access, and safety, Donabedian thought that medical quality training programs would quickly expand across the United States and that in 20 years, "clinical outcomes management" would attract thousands of physicians into this new field of population health care.

Now, some 18 years after these prophecies, we know that he was absolutely correct about the eventual dire need for professional accountability in health care quality, costs, and risk management. However, he greatly underestimated the lack of leadership by governments, the free-market system—and in certain instances, organized medicine and the medical education system—to provide the knowledge, training, and placement of medical quality physicians who would lead the medical quality movement into the 21st century. The serious gaps in quality accountability that are so well chronicled by eminent publications and distinguished institutions, such as the Institute of Medicine (National Academy of Sciences), are the result of this lack of leadership. Part of the quality gap in the US health care system is caused by the lack of adequate numbers of medical quality physicians to help integrate and account for the collective efforts of various formal and informal programs within national, state, and local health care services.

Instead of a large, well supported, and well integrated national medical specialty society that regularly contributes to the medical education curriculum, the current gaps are filled by a modest community of physician volunteers who lead the medical quality mission by example, with the hope that their efforts will eventually galvanize national and local leaders to bridge the huge quality chasm that wastes lives and precious resources every day. It is in this spirit of shared professional responsibility and commitment to the public good that this book has been brought to fruition.

I earnestly hope that this text will begin to address physicians' and other professionals' needs for current information about medical quality management principles, methods, programs, systems, and experiences. As such, this book represents an assessment of the "state of the nation" for quality management. I also trust that it will stimulate the formation of critically overdue and rarely adequately-funded medical education programs in quality management—especially in the area of endowed fellowship training.

Likewise, the American College of Medical Quality envisions this core curriculum in quality as a foundation for a meaningful, professionally and publicly recognized medical certification process. The current major drivers for medical quality—consumers, physicians, hospitals, payers, and health services researchers—need a common knowledge base for developing accountability for medical quality. Thus, the following chapters are a springboard for what the American College of Medical Quality sincerely hopes will be a greater fulfillment of its mission: to expand and promote the quality of health care that can be consistently provided to all citizens.

In a manner similar to Donabedian's organization of core knowledge into topical areas with established disciplines and publications, this book is organized into critical subject areas. The authors are all recognized leaders in their respective occupations; they have distinguished themselves as educators, researchers, writers, and missionaries in the medical quality movement. Given space limitations, no chapter can be considered comprehensive. Nevertheless, the reader should find this to be a highly credible basic text from which a sound initial working knowledge of medical quality management can be acquired. Individual chapters are noteworthy for the following:

1. Pelberg provides one of the most thorough published reviews of the key principles, methods, and proponents of quality in health care, especially over the past 25 years, which comprise the modern era of health care quality in the United States. The many practical, detailed, concise, and experience-based examples reinforce the depth and breadth of this *core* chapter in the core curriculum.

2. Silfen and Rosenblum provide an excellent summary of utilization management, including general approaches and methods, support systems, regulatory constructs, and common outcomes. The importance of realistic utilization management program objectives, design, qualified personnel, effective information and management systems, and evaluation methods are essential considerations in utilization accountability. Additionally, truly effective utilization management is always integrated into quality and risk management activities at every step in the overall health delivery process.

3. Ziegenfuss focuses on the ever-present interactive influences of an organization's leadership, human behavior, organizational structures, and management systems on quality outcomes. He describes some key evolutions in health care quality management and the progressive evolution of quality management through empirical measures of performance and collective responsibilities for organizational outcomes. Finally, he outlines the theories and principles that are relevant for the study and practice of quality management and describes several valuable applications of these principles.

4. Fetterolf and Braun make a number of critical points in their review of the economic, financial, and governmental issues affecting medical quality. They emphasize the importance of continually evaluating cost-quality interactions as a basis for improving performance, budgeting, and policymaking by health care organizations. Their discussion of the business and economic principles that are essential for medical quality professionals fulfills one of Donabedian's areas of emphasis. A particularly important point to consider is their view that quality management initiatives can be presented in economic terms through a variety of economic, clinical, administrative, operational, and social models. Notably, their many relevant points are elaborated in several instructive case studies that integrate the principles and promote critical thinking.

5. In 1986, Donabedian wrote about the world of paper files and elementary computer systems; Diamond expands Donabedian's study by describing the current world of global networks, micro-computing technologies, and increasingly sophisticated medical informatics programs. He reviews developments in evidence-based medicine, electronic medical records, and public and private data warehouse and analysis systems. He acknowledges that, for all of the sophisticated information technologies, the nation and its many disconnected health care organizations have failed to close many of the gaps that result in medical errors, poorly coordinated clinical decisionmaking, and frequently wasteful budgeting and planning processes. He underscores the continuing gaps and conflicts remaining because of a lack of national consensus for data definitions, standards, quality controls, and comprehensive integrated and critical quality data. Although current federal legislative and executive efforts—as well as some private efforts, such as the Leapfrog Group initiative—are encouraging, they remain largely disconnected and uneven in their impact, even if they are innovative and promising. Nevertheless, Diamond reminds us that inadequate data systems remain a major barrier to achieving national health quality aspirations.

6. Mislove provides an overview of important legislative, regulatory, and case law on which quality of care is based in various health care structures and processes. Notably, risk management from a legal perspective is often reactive and directed toward preventing adverse occurrences that impose serious financial and other liabilities on health care organizations and practitioners. From a quality management perspective, risk management in the future could and should serve as a source of quality improvement, and should therefore be fully integrated into quality and utilization management activities. Mislove also emphasizes the importance of legal protections for confidentiality in professional peer review activities and in patient privacy. Confidentiality is a cornerstone privilege in any democratic nation, but current government protections of privacy are sometimes at odds with the information access needed for quality improvement, prevention, disease management, and patient safety activities.

Zale focuses on the increasing application of medical ethics in a health care system that is increasingly driven by issues of economics, consumer demand, and availability of medical and information technologies. The complex situations that now routinely arise in individual and health policy decisions require more structured and standard approaches to ethical analysis and decision support for all those who collaborate in shared decisionmaking.

This book does not disappoint in its much anticipated arrival; it is filled with highly relevant references upon which thoughtful commentaries are consistently provided. It contains much in the way of experience, facts, and insights for both novice and seasoned health professionals who wish to understand the essentials of medical quality management. This book will take some time to read and will require even more time to digest its many important ideas, but each page will be instructive. So, please sit back and enjoy this minor version of a magnum opus on medical quality management. Then go and apply the information herein to improve the health care system in your community. In doing so, at whichever location or level of the health care system you may practice, we hope you will be inspired to take an *active lead* in the quality movement, so that all organizations involved in the health care system will follow you and the growing number of dedicated medical quality professionals who are helping to lead the improvements in health care quality in the United States.

References

1. Williamson JW. *Teaching Quality Assurance and Cost Containment in Health Care.* San Francisco: Jossey-Bass; 1982.

2. Williamson JW, Hudson JI, Nevins MM. *Principles of Quality Assurance and Cost Containment in Health Care.* San Francisco: Jossey-Bass; 1982.

3. Tobias RB, Ziegenfuss JT. *Quality Assurance and Utilization Review: Current Readings in Concept and Practice.* Sarasota, Florida: American Board of Quality Assurance and Utilization Review Physicians; 1987.

4. Stricker G, Rodriguez AR. *Handbook of Quality Assurance in Mental Health.* New York: Plenum; 1988.

5. Wilson L, Goldschmidt P. *Quality Management in Health Care.* Roseville, Australia: McGraw-Hill; 1995.

6. Claflin N, Hayden CT. *Guide To Quality Management, Eighth Edition.* Chicago: National Association for Healthcare Quality; 1998.

7. Kongstvedt PR, Plocher DW. *Best Practices in Medical Management.* Gaithersburg, Maryland: Aspen; 1998.

8. Lighter DE, Fair DC. *Principles and Methods of Quality Management in Health Care.* Gaithersburg, Maryland: Aspen; 2000.

9. Couch JB. *Health Care Quality Management for the 21st Century.* Tampa, Florida: American College of Physician Executives; 1991.

10. Donabedian A. *A Position Paper on the Future of ACURP.* Ann Arbor: University of Michigan; 1986.

ACKNOWLEDGMENTS

The American College of Medical Quality board of trustees acknowledges with appreciation the work of the following volunteer reviewers: George Beranek, MD, MBA; Paul Bronston, MD; Donald Casey, Jr., MD, MPH; Patricia Cholewka, EdD, MPA, MSN; Michael Corder, MD, MHA; Stephen Dorfman, MD; Scott Endsley, MD; Grant Lawless, MD, PharmD; Deborah Fuller, MHSA; Mark Granoff, MD, PhD, MPH; John Hinton, DO, MPH; George Martin, MD; Robert Masterson, DO, MBA; Thomas McBride, MD; Kenneth Patric, MD; Merhdad Shafa, MD, MMM; Dexter Shurney, MD, MBA, MPH; Otto Sieber, MD; and Hugo Velarde, MD.

ACMQ further acknowledges the exceptional contributions of James Ziegenfuss, Jr., PhD, project editor, and Mark Lyles, MD, project leader.

Thanks are also due to Bridget Brodie, ACMQ's executive vice president, who served as project manager and administrator.

CONTRIBUTORS

Joseph L. Braun, MD, JD, MBA

Joe Braun is a senior manager with PricewaterhouseCoopers' Healthcare Consulting Practice in Tampa, Florida. He has extensive experience working with medically related business, legal, and administrative issues on the provider and the payer's side. His focus is on process evaluation to improve efficiency, increase quality, reduce costs, and decrease the possibility of medical errors. He also has extensive experience with setting up clinical research programs, their structures, and their operations. He most recently worked at Aetna, Inc. as their national medical director for disability. Previously, he taught at George Washington University and has worked for Monsanto/Searle as their medical director. While living in Houston, he practiced law, specializing in health regulation and intellectual property. He received his MD from the University of Maryland, his JD from the University of Houston and is working on his PhD at George Washington University. His research areas are biotechnology, nanotechnology, and the future of medicine. Dr. Braun was a member of the American College of Medical Quality board of trustees from 2000 to 2004.

Louis H. Diamond, MB, ChB

Lou Diamond is vice president and medical director of Medstat, a health care information company that provides market intelligence and benchmark databases, decision support solutions, and research services for managing the cost and quality of health care. Dr. Diamond's expertise includes the use of health care information technologies, and methodologies for quality, and clinical performance measurement and improvement. His focus includes the use of knowledge management, business intelligence, and workflow process improvement techniques to drive quality improvement and cost reduction in our nation's health care system. He is also involved in the development of public policy through projects focused on patient safety, health system financing, physician payment reform, and quality measurement and reporting. Dr. Diamond received his medical degree in his native South Africa, where he was elected to fellowship in the College of Physicians. He has served as president of the

Medical Society of the District of Columbia as well as the Renal Physicians Association and now serves as RPA's representative to the AMA House of Delegates. Dr. Diamond was a Robert Wood Johnson health policy fellow and worked in the office of former Senate Majority Leader George Mitchell. He is a current member of the American College of Medical Quality board of trustees.

Donald E. Fetterolf, MD, MBA

Don Fetterolf is vice president and chief medical officer for Highmark Blue Cross Blue Shield in Pittsburgh, with operating responsibilities for medical directors, quality management, and strategic physician services and with oversight responsibilities involving indemnity, PPO, HMO, point of service, and Medicare business. He is the creator and former medical director of Highmark's medical informatics department. Dr. Fetterolf received his MD degree and his MBA, as well as dual undergraduate degrees in chemistry and biochemistry, from the University of Pennsylvania in Philadelphia. He is currently a clinical assistant professor of medicine at the University of Pittsburgh Medical Center and at Temple University School of Medicine. He is on the teaching faculty at Duquesne University. Dr. Fetterolf is a member of the American College of Medical Quality board of trustees and on the editorial boards of several journals including the *American Journal of Medical Quality* and *Disease Management*. In the past, he served as an internist in private practice for 12 years. Prior managed care experience includes having been medical director for a 150,000 member health network PPO, where he had also functioned as chairman of the board and its president/CEO, and president of a hospital PHO. He currently serves as a member of the technical advisory group for the Pennsylvania Health Care Cost Containment Council.

Joseph A. Mislove, JD, MBA

Joe Mislove is chief counsel for compliance and regulatory affairs at Schaller Anderson, a national health care management and consulting company based in Phoenix, where he directs compliance activities and counsels management on health care regulatory issues. He has practiced health care law since 1989 in both private practice and as in-house counsel. Prior to joining Schaller Anderson, Mr. Mislove was a member of Coppersmith Gordon Schermer Owens and Nelson P.L.C., a Phoenix law firm with a nationally recognized expertise in health care law. Mr. Mislove has written and lectured extensively on health care law topics, including regulation of claim payment practices, peer review, managed care contracting, the National Practitioner and the Healthcare Integrity and Protection Data Banks, medical record confidentiality, sentinel events under JCAHO, and EMTALA. He received BS and MBA degrees from Arizona State University in 1981 and 1986, respectively, and his JD degree from the University of Arizona in 1986. He is a member of the American Health Lawyers Association and an executive committee member of the Arizona Association of Health Care Lawyers, serving as president of the latter organization from 1996 to 1997.

Arthur L. Pelberg, MD, MPA

Arthur Pelberg is president and chief medical officer of Schaller Anderson, a national health care management and consulting company based in Phoenix. He directs the CEOs and medical directors of the managed care organizations administered by Schaller Anderson affiliates and is responsible for the oversight of medical management, including quality and utilization systems. Before joining Schaller Anderson he was in medical practice for more than 19 years and was corporate medical director for an HMO and an ambulatory and emergency care center. Dr. Pelberg earned his medical degree from Temple University and his master's degree in public administration from Pennsylvania State University. He is board certified in internal medicine and completed a fellowship in quality management at the Pennsylvania State University College of Medicine. He is a member of the Area Advisory Committee for the Medicare Competitive Bid Project and has been a reviewer for the National Committee for Quality Assurance. In addition, he was a general medical officer and service unit director in the Public Health Service, Indian Health Service in Arizona. Dr. Pelberg is a fellow of the American College of Medical Quality as well as a past president and current board member. He has published articles in peer-reviewed journals and frequently lectures and consults at national and regional seminars related to managed care and medical management.

Alex R. Rodriguez, MD

Alex Rodriguez is executive vice president and chief medical officer of Magellan Health Services in Farmington, Connecticut. He formerly was chief medical officer of two other national managed care organizations, and has served as medical director and chief of quality assurance for CHAMPUS (Department of Defense) and as special assistant to the Secretary of the U.S. Department of Health and Human Services. He has been a member of the boards of the Utilization Review Accreditation Commission and Disease Management Association of America, and has been active in the National Committee on Quality Assurance as a surveyor and chair of the Behavioral Health Accreditation and Performance Measurement Committee. Dr. Rodriguez is a graduate of Emory University's School of Medicine and completed his medical training at the University of California, San Francisco. Board certified in psychiatry and medical management, he has maintained a continuous medical practice in the Naval Reserve, where he has also served in a number of command leadership positions. He has been on the faculty at Yale School of Medicine since 1987, and previously taught at the medical schools at the University of California, University of Colorado, and Uniformed Services University of the Health Sciences. He has published numerous articles and book chapters, and is the co-author and editor of *Quality Assurance in Mental Health*. Dr. Rodriguez is a former president of the American College of Medical Quality, and has served as the literature review editor of the *American Journal of Medical Quality* since its inception in 1985.

Ralph H Rosenblum, Jr., DDS, MHA

Ralph Rosenblum is currently the dental chief and manager of dental services for the Ohio State University Student Health Services. He is responsible for the operation of the service, quality mandates, and JCAHO certification. He is also a medical quality consultant and a practicing clinician. Dr. Rosenblum has been both associate medical director and director of dental programs for United HealthCare Corporation. He has also participated in many voluntary quality activities as a member of boards of directors, executive committees, task forces, and community project activities since 1972. He has published many articles and given numerous seminar presentations, as well as having been awarded Honorable Mention for Excellence in Dental Journalism from the International College of Dentists and the 2005 Service Award from the American College of Medical Quality in recognition of his long-time editorship of the ACMQ newsletter. Dr. Rosenblum received his bachelor's degree in1967 from Miami University of Ohio, his DDS from the Ohio State University College of Dentistry in 1972, and his master's degree in health care administration from Seton Hall University in 2000.

Eric Z. Silfen, MD, MHSA

Eric Silfen is post-doctoral fellow and director of executive programs in the Department of Biomedical Informatics at Columbia University. He is also a trustee and partner at Chironet, LLC, an Internet health care knowledge management firm that uses proprietary software to support the collection, tracking, and trending of patient-level data. He was previously chief medical officer at St. Charles Hospital and Rehabilitation Center in Port Jefferson, New York and chief medical officer at HCA Reston Hospital Center in Virginia. Dr. Silfen earned his medical degree at Georgetown University School of Medicine and his master of science in health administration from the Medical College of Virginia, where he was adjunct associate professor for six years in the Department of Health Administration. He is board certified in both emergency medicine and internal medicine and completed residencies in both specialties at Georgetown University School of Medicine. Dr. Silfen has published extensively and presented lectures nationwide. He is currently president-elect of the American College of Medical Quality.

Jeffrey Zale, MD, MPH

Jeff Zale is currently the medical director for quality assurance at the Delmarva Foundation, the Maryland and District of Columbia quality improvement organization (QIO). His major responsibilities include quality assurance and peer review activities in addition to roles in the area of external quality review of Medicaid and Medicare managed care plans. He has had over 20 years of experience in managed care as a clinician and medical director involved with medical management, including utilization management, peer review, credentialing and quality assurance, and improvement. Prior to serving as medical director at a large for-profit managed care plan serving Medicare, Medicaid, and commercial populations, he functioned in a number of clinical and administrative roles in a large medical group affiliated with Johns Hopkins. He is board certified in family practice and has practiced in both an office-based environment and an emergency department.

James T. Ziegenfuss, Jr., PhD

Jim Ziegenfuss is professor of management and health care systems in the graduate programs in health and public administration, at the School of Public Affairs at Pennsylvania State University. He teaches graduate courses in health care quality management, health care systems, strategic planning, organization behavior, and organization and management problem solving. Professor Ziegenfuss holds the PhD in social systems sciences from the Wharton School of the University of Pennsylvania, master's degrees in psychology (Temple) and public administration (Penn State) and a bachelor's degree in English (University of Maryland). At the Penn State Medical College, he is adjunct professor of medicine, active in education and research. Dr. Ziegenfuss has written over 100 articles for journals and conferences, authored 10 books and edited 4 books. His most recent works include *Portable Health Administration* (2004) and *Organization and Management Problem Solving: A Systems and Consulting Approach* (2002). He has been Associate Editor of the *American Journal of Medical Quality* since 1989. Professor Ziegenfuss' current interests are the topics of quality management, strategic planning, and the design of customer-friendly organizations. A consultant to both the public and private sectors, his education, research, and consulting has been supported by more than 70 organizations including medical schools, associations, hospitals, and non-profit organizations.

Chapter 1

QUALITY MANAGEMENT PRINCIPLES AND PRACTICES

Arthur L. Pelberg, MD, MPA

Introduction

This chapter introduces quality management theories and practices that have evolved over the past 25 years; it does not attempt to provide an exhaustive history of theory and practice. Instead, it highlights some themes that have marked the progress of the field over recent decades. It also addresses points of philosophy and practice that characterize the field today.

The chapter is organized around five key questions:

- How did we arrive at the current state of quality management?
- What is the purpose and philosophy of quality management?
- What are the approaches, methods, and procedures of quality management?
- What are the expected outcomes of quality management activities?
- What organizations are involved in quality management?

The Quality Management Movement to the Present

In 1914, Codman challenged hospitals and physicians to take responsibility for the outcomes of their patients.[1] The health care industry has taken some time to respond to this challenge. In the 1960s, Donabedian created the structure, process, and outcome paradigm for assessing quality in health care.[2] Accrediting bodies, such as the National Committee for Quality Assurance (NCQA) and the Joint Commission for the Accreditation of Health Organizations (JCAHO), have long recognized the importance of process variables and are increasingly incorporating outcome assessment into their activities.

In the 1980s and 1990s, Berwick identified new approaches to quality improvement for health care, including continuous quality improvement (CQI) and total quality management (TQM), by introducing the management ideas of Juran,[3] Deming,[4] and Crosby.[5] In 1998, Chassin and Galvin characterized the problems of overuse,

1

underuse, and misuse in medicine and called attention to the variation in the practice of medicine and to the suboptimal patient outcomes associated with this variation.[6]

The history of quality management is best told by highlighting some key developments. Nine topics, explored in subsequent subsections, nicely summarize the history of quality management over the past 80 years or so: early efforts, clinical quality focus, conceptual foundations, professional autonomy, parallel industrial quality efforts, the movement to total quality, the Malcolm Baldrige Quality Awards, support system developments, and the recent Institute of Medicine studies.

An Early Start

Physicians did not just arrive at an interest in quality at the close of the 20th century. Codman recognized the need to examine the outcomes of his surgical work nearly 100 years ago, in 1914. It has taken health care close to 100 years to include the idea of quality in health care to become part of the mainstream of medicine.

Clinical Quality Assurance

After Codman's early efforts, the next 60 to 70 years focused mostly on clinical activities of clinical teams: transactions between physicians and patients in clinics, hospitals, and practices. The structure sought to identify deficient practitioners and mandate "improvements," such as punishments, or even weeding out those recalcitrant clinicians who refused to change. The focus on clinical activities did not recognize the contribution of other organizational characteristics, which include leadership, resources, information systems, and communication patterns among teams. The patient's consideration of quality was certainly not included; it was a narrow, "policing-oriented" philosophy that focused on the providers of care, ferreting out the "bad apples."

Conceptual Foundations of Quality Management

During the latter half of the 20th century, the initial struggle involved a conceptual base to open the field. Early researchers such as Codman had little theoretical and conceptual base on which to build. The work of Avedis Donabedian had enormous influence, to the extent that he is often thought of as the modern founder and leader of the quality management field.[2] His famous presentation of the quality management task as a function of understanding the stages of structure, process, and outcome had a widespread national and international impact after its publication in the 1960s. This pioneering presentation remains the dominant work on the purpose and process of the quality management effort. It identifies the relationships between process and outcome and how they are linked to improved patient outcomes. Donabedian's work is based on recognizing the values of the physician-patient relationship and the uniqueness of the medical and health care challenge of diversity of patient demands. His work has also helped establish the systems approach to health care quality and its studies.

Autonomy of Professionals

During much of this development period, professionals led the work in quality assurance—work mostly divided by medical discipline. Each professional discipline was expected to monitor the quality and safety of its particular field and was thus given autonomy from "outside examiners." Professionals tended to believe that they provided high-quality care "each time, to every patient." In the 1980s and 1990s, various stakeholders, such as purchasers, regulators, patients, and advocates, began to call for a more open examination of the quality of care. During these two decades, professionals experienced a gradual erosion of their autonomous quality control efforts. It was not enough to know that professionals were monitoring their own work; others wanted to see the data. This trend led the US Office of the Vice President to convene a Quality Forum Planning Committee to develop a National Forum for Health Care Quality Measurement and Reporting, which has become the National Quality Forum (NQF).

The Parallel Industrial Quality Track

During these quality improvement efforts in the medical field, people in industry were exploring the potential contribution of quality improvement efforts in their fields. In the 1980s and 1990s, the work of Crosby,[5] Juran,[3] and Deming[4] became well known in manufacturing across the United States. This work brought attention to systems design, process controls, and the involvement of the entire work force.

This brief history would be incomplete without describing the contribution of Edwards Deming and his industrial approach to quality management. Deming's main contribution is well represented by the 14 points of his philosophy, which define technical procedure and Deming's philosophy of intervention:

1. Create constancy of purpose.
2. Adopt a new philosophy.
3. Cease dependence on inspection.
4. Cease awarding business on the basis of price alone.
5. Improve continuously and forever.
6. Institute training and retraining on the job.
7. Adopt an institute leadership.
8. Drive out fear.
9. Break down barriers between staff members.
10. Eliminate slogans, exhortations, and targets for the workforce.
11. Eliminate numerical quotas for workers and numerical goals for managers.
12. Remove barriers that rob people of pride in workmanship.
13. Institute a vigorous program of education and self-improvement.
14. Put everybody in the organization to work on the transformation.

These points, which are widely recognized in medical and industrial circles, are both principles of his approach and guidelines for the quality management leaders whom Deming trained and encouraged. Many of the principles now guide medical quality efforts.

Deming's 14 points constituted a second conceptual development that both followed and pushed the Donabedian model. Quality management was redefined as not just a technical, clinical exercise but also an issue of culture and values, psychological climate, leadership and values, and another "mental model" of the improvement process.[4]

From Clinical Quality Management to Total Organization Quality Management

The implementation of the industrial model outside health care was widespread. Many executives served on hospital and health system boards, using those positions to push medical quality leaders to look beyond the boundaries of clinical quality assurance. Now the targets for improvement could include all aspects of the health care organization, from leadership style and behavior, to the presence of information system support, to the level of collaboration between departments and disciplines. Clinical quality management was now seen as part of "total quality management" (TQM), defined as the continuous effort to improve every aspect of the organization's operations—also known as continuous quality improvement (CQI). An example is the Leapfrog program, which has identified three specific ways to improve the quality of in-patient hospital care and is supported by purchasers of health care. These process changes are: (1) using hospitals that perform a specific number of procedures, (2) using intensivists in Intensive Care Units, and (3) having electronic order entry for physicians.

Malcolm Baldrige Quality Awards

The Malcolm Baldrige Quality Awards were started for the industrial sector in 1987 under Public Law 100-107. These awards, which were first given in 1988, recognize organizations that meet specific quality standards. These national awards did much to encourage thinking about quality management in every aspect of business and industry. Recognizing outstanding quality took on great symbolic importance nationally. By emphasizing the seven areas of the awards' criteria (leadership; strategic planning; focus on patients, other customers, and markets; information and analysis; staff focus; process management; and organizational performance results), the awards pushed the thinking of quality management leaders to encompass a broader perspective of the quality target—literally, any and all aspects of the organization.

Information Systems Support

The last several decades of the 20th century have also seen enormous progress in the development of information systems. These systems are needed to obtain the data of health care so that quality processes can be applied to decrease variations and improve outcomes.

Institute of Medicine Reports and Other Studies

In the last 10 years, a series of studies on the scope and prevalence of medical errors has drawn much attention and has contributed to a renewed interest in quality.[7] These studies have caused distress and have motivated change. In 1998, Chassin and Galvin reported that large numbers of medical errors were occurring in health care.[6] These errors were not caused by a particular payment system because the errors were documented across managed care and fee-for-service providers. Other researchers have found the error rate in medicine to be between 12% and 30%. Most attention has been focused on medication errors. By some estimates, medication errors account for almost 40% of all adverse patient outcomes.[7] Other types of errors also deserve attention: surgical errors, diagnostic errors, and the inappropriate use of hospital services. Nonstandard processes of care, lack of a systems approach, and inadequate management information systems are now known to contribute to large variations in care and adverse patient outcomes. In 1999, Corrigan and Donaldson estimated that at least 75,000 people die from medical errors every year. Under their editorship, the Institute of Medicine (IOM) of the National Academies published *To Err Is Human: Building a Safer Health System* in 2000.[7] The report identified the systems that needed to be developed to decrease the number of medical errors in the United States. In *Crossing the Quality Chasm: A New Health System for the 21st Century*,[8] the IOM defined the state of the quality problem, offered recommendations for improvements, and outlined specific targets that would contribute to nationwide improvements.

The Purpose and Philosophy of Quality Management

The purpose and philosophy of quality management has evolved from an orientation toward policing (finding "bad apples" among primarily excellent physicians, nurses, and clinical teams) to the use of quality management as a tool for continuous development of high performance.

Quality management can be thought of as having three aspects:

1. A means of *accountability* for the use of clinical and physical resources in the care of patients.
2. An effort to *continuously develop and improve* the services provided to patients by care teams throughout the organization and the community.
3. A mechanism to improve the *clinical outcomes of patients* as defined by the patient and the health care system.

The early focus of quality measurement was on a narrow definition of the target—clinical medical services only. However, as physicians gained experience in their efforts to improve clinical quality assurance, many realized that the rest of the organization also contributed to the success or failure of clinical transactions. For example, members of the clinical team in an operating room realized that, although they did an outstanding job of attending to the surgical needs of the patient, recovery in a hospital bed—somewhere in the hospital—was beyond their control. They realized, for instance, that a shortage of nurses could cause a lack of attention to the care needs of the patient, and that decisions by hospital administrators to lay off nurses, mandate double shifts for nurses' work, or deny nurses opportunities to participate in strategic decisions could all hinder a hospital's ability to recruit and retain nurses. Therefore, they acknowledged that the fine work done by the clinical team in the operating room could be undercut by decisions made by hospital administrators who were far removed from the direct clinical action.

Because the focus of quality management has broadened, quality management programs currently tend to include as targets *both clinical and organizational structures and processes* that lead to improved outcomes (i.e., the traditional clinical-medical focus of quality assurance and the more recent interest in developing high-performance organizations through total quality management). High-performance organizations provide the best outcomes for the patient through the use of system integration, including continuous quality improvement (CQI) and total quality management (TQM).

An example will show how the philosophy of quality management is applied in the health care setting. At a 15-year-old trauma center in a 475-bed urban hospital, the medical director and his staff decided that continuous quality improvement would add value to their services. Quality management leaders answered their inquiries about continuous quality improvement in light of the current philosophy of quality management, which is summarized in the following eight points:

1. *Systems thinking.* Quality management leaders view quality as enacted in a set of interlocking systems: the technology of diagnosis and treatment, the structure of incentives, the psychological climate, and the culture of high performance. Quality is an outcome of coordinated systems. Each system is interdependent; none is an independent force for quality. Interventions to improve quality are thus necessarily multidimensional. When the trauma staff considered at their center the interdependence of systems, they realized that they would have to include the pre-hospital emergency service teams in their quality improvement work. Although the teams are *outside* the hospital system, they are *within* the patient's system of trauma care services.

2. *Micro and macro orientation.* Quality is assessed and improved by making decisions at the operating service level (e.g., at the level of an operating-room team), which is sometimes called the *micro level*. Quality can also be assessed and improved by making strategic decisions at the *macro level* (e.g., by deciding to drop a trauma service because the hospital is unable to recruit, retain, and pay for the 24-hour-a-day surgical team needed to staff the unit). Quality management philosophy requires operating teams and institutional leaders to make decisions that support quality at the macro and micro levels of the organization. The trauma center staff recognized a need to focus on two levels: the speed with which clinical teams responded to incoming patients (micro level), and strategic concerns that arose from the hospital's inability to fund and recruit the full staff needed to cover all shifts adequately (macro level). The trauma center staff realized that resources were a hospital-wide issue, not just a trauma center issue.

3. *Patient-focused orientation.* The attention to redesign is based on a "patient first" orientation that forces the institution to alter processes and structures to support patient needs, convenience, and confidentiality. Patients are often used in quality improvement redesign efforts to ensure that their feedback is fully heard, and they are also used in the diagnosis-planning-action-evaluation improvement cycle. In the trauma center, the primary interests of the staff should be to consider the clinical pathways taken by various types of patients and to increase the scope, response time, and depth of services to patients who have immediate and significant care needs.

4. *Use of metrics, data, and information in the quality management processes.* In every aspect of the quality improvement effort, data and facts are used along with professional judgment and patient feedback. Collecting information about the nature of the problem, the extent of variation and control, benchmark standards, and the effect of the changes is a core component of the quality improvement process. In the trauma center, collecting and analyzing information on the flow of patients was not an accustomed activity, even though some data were available. Response times, mortality, and return to surgery were routinely tracked, but not in the context of a search for improved opportunities and redesign.

5. *Recognition of multiple causes and co-producers.* Following on the systems thinking concept, all quality deficiencies are thought to have multiple causes. Because poor quality is "co-produced," interventions designed to improve systems and teams must also have sets of actions that will serve to "co-produce" improvements. As the trauma center team began to examine sample cases, they saw that some delays in providing care were issues of communication and coordination, whereas other delays arose from competing duties of the staff. They realized that redesign would require participation by multiple stakeholders and changes in several systems at once, and that the changes in the systems would have to be narrow in scope and instituted rapidly. They decided that the system changes that produced improved outcomes would be continued, and those that did not would be discarded and new ones tried. Their realization led to the concept of rapid or short-cycle change, instead of the traditional quality management program in which one idea for change was implemented and measured over a long period of time.

6. *Participation and empowerment of the workforce.* Quality management leaders believe that improvement will result from engaging the workforce and from allowing participation in the quality effort by literally "everyone in the organization," especially physicians.[9] All workers—clinical, administrative, and support personnel—must feel that they can take action to identify and correct design and process flaws, and that they are "allowed and encouraged" to point to opportunities for improvement. The success of the quality management program depends not only on workforce em-

powerment but also on support from the highest levels of the organization. This support must be a philosophical "buy in" as well as a resource commitment.

When the trauma center staff proposed some changes that would affect administrative routines and resource levels, hospital administrators initially tabled the ideas. After some pestering, the administrators suggested that the trauma clinical staff stay within its area of expertise—clinical services to patients—and leave redesign to the hospital team.

7. *Continuous individual and organizational development as the goal.* Currently, quality management philosophy views continuous individual and organizational development as the goal. Recognizing that quality management must incorporate both micro and macro targets—clinical teams as well as organization-wide strategic decisions—quality management leaders view the mission as a never-ending task, a continuous striving to be better next year than this year in all aspects of direct patient care and outcomes, and in every aspect of administrative and support services.

Several trauma center staff members were aware that trauma centers in San Diego, Baltimore, and Philadelphia were the leaders in services and organization. They proposed a benchmarking study of these leading programs to gain a better understanding of the structures and processes by which these programs achieved their high performance status. Participants in the study were "educated" about new designs, and several of these designs were put into place (organizational development). Figure 1–1 shows the specific concepts of CQI that have been discussed in the trauma example. The diagram drills down to specific components of quality improvement.

8. *An external and internal orientation.* Many organizations were initially "dragged to the quality improvement table " by external regulatory organizations. The perception was that quality was im-

Figure 1–1   Concepts of Total Quality Management

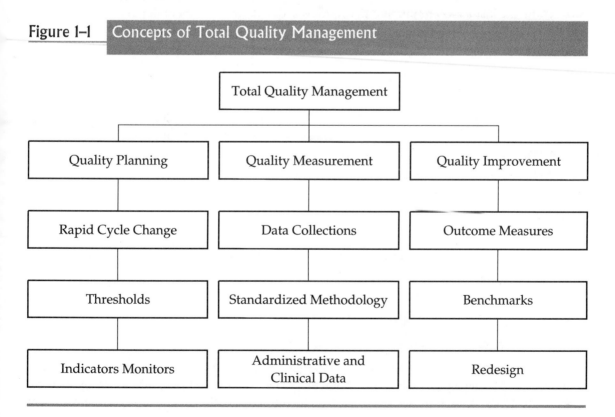

portant because it was a regulatory requirement (i.e., mandated). Others saw quality improvement as an important goal for the organization's future success—a way to build competitiveness, a desirable goal for patient care irrespective of mandates, and a personal value of the culture of clinicians and administrators. Currently, many leaders view quality as not just a regulatory necessity, but a part of their personal and organizational mission. Their intent is to push their own internal quality interests further and faster than is required by regulators. Continuous improvement is now an "internally" generated mission.

In the trauma center, most staff members had spent years grumbling about the Trauma Center Accreditation Process, which was cumbersome and time-consuming, and they resented the drain on their clinical time. However, as they gained a better understanding of the quality philosophy, they saw the accreditation as a part of the package of strategies for increasing quality throughout the center. Eventually, they took pride in the comprehensiveness of their internal quality effort, going well beyond external demands. Their internal quality improvement process eventually supplanted the external quality requirements of accreditation in power and scope.

These eight themes are fairly well recognized by quality management leaders. They are less well understood by individual clinicians and clinical teams, many of whom still think of modern quality management as characterized by the policing philosophy of early clinical quality assurance.

Modern quality management leaders are systems thinkers, attending to both operating and strategic-level issues that concern quality. These quality management leaders put patients first, use data and information to examine and respond to problems, and rely on the participation of the entire workforce. They constantly seek changes that will *co-produce* improvement in a continuous cycle. Although outside regulators may check on the quality of care, the concerns of "outsiders" are dwarfed by the insiders' commitment to continuous quality improvement of patient care systems and the outcomes they produce.

Methods and Procedures

The methods and procedures used in quality management have nine critical aspects, which are described in subsequent subsections:

1. Quality management plans and work plans
2. Levels of inquiry and quality management
3. Baseline assessment and benchmarking
4. Quality improvement process steps
5. Measurement challenges
6. Information systems support: indicators and monitors
7. Methods and tools
8. Outcomes assessment
9. Integrated approaches

Quality Management Plans and Work Plans

Most organizations use a planning process to initiate the quality management program and to design total quality management activities. Sometimes the organization plan developed by medical and administrative leaders at the executive level incorporates both strategic decisions and clinical quality efforts at the operating team level. At other times, strategic and operating plans are semi- or completely autonomous. Planning is more effective when the entire organization's intention to stimulate and support continuous organization-wide quality improvement is linked with the individual clinical team's work to improve quality in patient care (e.g, in the operating room, in radiology, in pediatrics, and in the admissions process).

Quality management planning by senior medical and administrative leaders signals that the organization regards quality as an important strategic issue. The quality plan recognizes that advocacy groups, regulators, competitors, and clients demand information on quality levels and quality improvement initiatives.

Operational quality work plans are developed by clinical teams to further their specific quality initiatives (e.g., a discharge process may be improved by examining the flow of reports from radiology to the clinical units, or studying the response time in the trauma center); such an improvement is considered to be the purview of the clinical quality improvement program.

Most processes for quality management planning include the following steps:

1. Declaring an intention to plan for quality improvement and agreeing on a process
2. Defining present levels of quality, including assessments of industry standards, competitor quality levels, and internal quality levels
3. Having a vision and design for the desired quality outcomes
4. Comparing the quality outcomes as desired with the quality at present, including specifically identifying the gaps between present and future opportunities for improvement
5. Choosing strategies and actions designed to enhance quality
6. Implementing a process for taking action
7. Devising an evaluation process and choosing a point in time for checking progress

Depending on the philosophical orientation of the quality leaders, work plans are more or less quantitative, although most plans have specific indicators by which quality progress can be measured. Some quality improvement plans are elaborate and "paper-intensive." Others are lean, and progress is mostly tracked orally in meetings by senior leaders and clinical teams.

Plans for a quality improvement effort can be structured by answering a series of questions:

1. What is the general approach and philosophy of quality management, and what are potential areas for improvement in data collection, measurement, and outcome evaluation? Are policies established, and is there a written plan for quality improvement?
2. How can improvement be measured?
3. What is the relationship of the quality program to top management, including reporting line and authority base? What is the culture of the organization concerning quality?
4. Who is the quality leader, and what is his or her rank, professional field, and training? (Having the "buy-in" of clinical leaders in the organization greatly enhances the acceptance and success of the quality management program.) What is the expense for the quality leader?
5. What is the structure of the quality program (advisory committee or council; number and type of quality teams)? (The structure should be formalized and accepted by the organization, with reporting to an appropriate organizational level.)
6. What is the quality improvement model, including procedures, techniques, and methods; quantitative and qualitative orientation; accomplishments; pilots; computer support; and

staff participants? (Metrics and methodologies must be well-established and identified for the program to be accepted.)

7. Who is staffing the program (numbers, types, roles)? What are the roles of the staff members in the organization?

8. What is the start-up process (initial activities and timelines)? Are the resources sufficient to launch the program?

9. Will external assistance be used (design consultants, process advisors, trainers)?

10. What are the direct and indirect costs (return on investment; cost of poor quality)? (These costs can be financial, clinical, or operational.)

11. How will the program be evaluated and controlled (periodic review; progress assessment)? (The organization needs to know how the program will be measured and how the results will be evaluated. There should be no surprises or tampering with the outcomes.)

Both strategic-level and operating-level plans are well served when detailed answers to the above questions are given. The answers should include specific monitors, metrics, and methodologies to document outcomes.

Answering all of these questions leads to three work tools: (1) the quality management plan, which usually identifies the general concepts of the quality management program and how it will operate over a period of time; (2) a work plan that identifies specific time lines, responsible parties, and clinical studies that operate under the quality management plan; and (3) an evaluation of the quality management plan and work plan. A table of contents for a quality management plan is shown in Table 1–1. A work plan for the program is displayed in Table 1–2, and an evaluation form is shown in Table 1–3.

Levels of Inquiry and Quality Management

Quality management leaders may attend to several levels of quality focus or inquiry: individual, team, unit, organization, and community. In large, comprehensive quality management programs, quality efforts include activities at each of these levels—clinical activities at the operating service level; team activities in a unit such as the cardiac or transplant care unit; organization-wide activities, such as the public launch of hospital-wide quality improvement; and outwardly directed community activities designed to improve quality of care delivered to a population or a community, such as the health communities movement.

The more ambitious the quality effort (i.e., the more levels of quality improvement focus), the greater is the need for organization-wide support and resources. For example, an individual clinical team could, on its own, initiate quality improvement processes that address its particular clinical transactions (e.g., what happens to the patient in the trauma care unit during the first 15 minutes after the patient's arrival). This quality diagnosis and improvement activity can be autonomously supported and encouraged by the leaders of the trauma center and by the clinicians, without the need for organization-wide support. However, an effort to extend the trauma team's pilot initiative in clinical quality improvement to other aspects of the surgical department, to the hospital at large, and outwardly toward the community (e.g., improvement of the pre-hospital emergency service system) is larger in scale and intent, and needs wider support.

Philosophically, quality management leaders believe that quality improvement will be achieved when all levels are attended to. In simple terms, the responsibility of quality management

| Table 1–1 | Table of Contents for a Quality Management Plan (QMP) |

1. Policy Statement
2. Program Accountability
3. Purpose
4. Goals
5. Objectives
6. Scope
7. Chief Medical Officer
8. Quality Management Work Plan
9. Committee Structure
10. Quality Management Oversight Committee (QMOC)
11. Quality Management Committee (QMC)
12. Credentialing Committee
13. Pharmacy and Therapeutics Committee
14. Annual Plan Evaluation and Revisions
15. Quality Management Department
16. Integration
17. Peer Review
18. Credential/Re-credential
19. Quality, Risk, and Utilization Management Screening and Referrals
20. Medical Record Review
21. Practitioner and Provider Contracting
22. Review, Monitoring, and Evaluation of Health Plan Activities
23. Performance Standards and Regulatory Compliance
24. Clinical Practice Guidelines
25. Indicators
26. Outcomes
27. Medical Studies/Patient Safety
28. Accessibility of Services
29. Continuity of Care
30. Satisfaction Surveys
31. Availability of Practitioners and Providers
32. Delegation Oversight
33. Conflict of Interest
34. Confidentiality Statement
35. Documentation and Retention of Records
36. Reconsideration of Appeals and Grievances

and improvement rests not just with the quality management department, but also with other clinical, financial, and operational units of the health care organization. Quality management and improvement must be an integrated program throughout the organization.

Baseline Assessment and Benchmarking

Almost all quality improvement programs begin with an assessment of the quality in the organization in its current state, which is known as a *baseline assessment*. To allow quality improvements toward a desirable quality outcome to be tracked, the starting point at the individual, team, unit, organization, or community level must be known. Baseline assessments use many types of quantitative and qualitative measures as indicators, and allow a supporting analysis and an eventual

Table 1-2 Corporate Template for a Quality Management Work Plan

Activity/Strategies (A)	Purpose/Objective; Action Taken (B)	Measurement/ Indicator (C)	Performance Goal/ Benchmark (D)	Responsible/ Reporting Party (E)	Committee Reporting (F)	Target Date (G)	Completion Date (H)	Outcome of Activity (I)
1 Administration: approval, QM program description, utilization management (UM) program description, QM work plan, and QM evaluation	To assure approval of the QM plan, UM plan, QM work plan, and evaluation	Approval of QM plan, UM plan, QM work plan, and evaluation	N/A	Chief Medical Officer (CMO), director of Quality Management (QM), manager of QM	Quality Management Oversight Committee (QMOC)			
2 Credentialing: improve timeliness of credentialing/ re-credentialing	To complete the initial credentialing process in ≤ 90 days	Current credentials of all MDs, DOs, DDSs, DMDs, DCs DPMs, BHPs	100% timely Re-credentialed every 3 years— 90% timely	Director of QM				
	To complete the re-credentialing process on or before the re-credentialing due date							
Organizational providers: • Home health agencies • Hospitals • Skilled nursing facilities • Nursing homes • Free-standing surgical centers • Behavioral health facilities	Pre-contract review and every 3 years		100% timely					

					QM manager
3	Delegation	To ensure all plan standards related to delegation functions are met	Delegation monitoring	Pre-assessment 100% complete	
			Percentage of compliance with initial and ongoing delegated requirements	Standards compliance at pre-assessment 90%	
				100% complete	
				Standards compliance at annual audit 90%	
4	Population analysis	To evaluate plan population mix	Analyze member population by sex and age		
		Evaluate provider network	No. of primary health providers (PHPs) and specialty health providers (SHPs)		

QM = quality management
UM = utilization management

Table 1-3 Evaluation Tool for a Quality Management Plan

Activity/ Strategies	Purpose/ Objective/ Action Taken	Measurement/ Indicator	Performance Goal/Benchmark Met/Not Met	Trending 2004	Trending 2005	Trending 2006	Target Date	Completion Date	Barriers

judgment to be made about the status of medical quality at that point in time. In Table 1–4, a baseline assessment is shown for a group of patients with diabetes whose hemoglobin (Hg) A1c levels were evaluated in year one. This evaluation was used for designing a quality improvement project and for determining the change in HgA1c levels after one year of intervention.

Quality improvement plans also include *benchmarking*. As part of an effort to determine the current status of quality in the team or organization, quality improvement team members may study the quality of competitors, peer organizations, and even organizations outside the health care industry, and may examine professional societies' standards.

Benchmarking has been used to identify best practices and to bring performance and outcomes to the best practice level.[10] The five basic steps for benchmarking are: (1) identifying benchmarking measures, (2) designing a data collection method and gathering data, (3) comparing the results with

| Table 1–4 | Baseline Assessment: Hemoglobin A1c Levels at Baseline and After a One-Year Intervention for 212 Patients with Diabetes |

Member interventions:
☐ Applied program
— Stratification of diabetic population
— Special needs case management
— Outreach activities and education
☐ Referrals to employer program

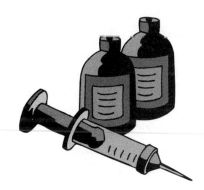

Provider interventions:
☐ Contacted physician and coordinated information
☐ Sponsored a physician education program

Member outcome:
☐ Improved diabetes control
— Lowered hemoglobin A1c

Direct cost savings:
☐ Reduced hospital readmission rate for diabetes

	Hemoglobin A1c Levels	
	Year 1	**Year 2**
N	212	212
Median	7.30%	7.10%
Average	7.62%	7.39%
% of Patients with Values < 7.5%	54.7%	60.8%
% of Patients with Values > 9.5%	16.5%	11.3%

a standard and determining the gap in performance, (4) identifying the practices needed to improve performance, and (5) determining resources needed to implement the practices. An Achievable Benchmark of Care (ABC), as identified by Kiefe et al.,[11] is produced by benchmarks that: (1) are measurable and attainable, (2) are based on the performance of the highest performers, and (3) provide an appropriate number of cases for analysis.

In short, the benchmarking effort is a search for the best practices that will support high-performance, high-quality care delivery. Benchmarking is often thought of as directed at competitors (i.e., team members need to know the level of quality against which they are competing). But benchmarking may also be directed at processes in other industries similar to those in the health care services (e.g., determining how quickly airline teams are able to prepare airplanes for departure after landing, just as teams clean and prepare operating rooms for the next patient).

Dean and Evans[12] gave an outstanding presentation of the benchmarking process in 1994, describing it as follows:

1. *Determine which functions to benchmark.* These should have a significant impact on business performance and key dimensions of competitiveness. If quick response is an important dimension of competitive advantage, then potential benchmark processes would include order processing, purchasing, production planning, and product distribution. There should also be an indication that the potential for improvement exists.

2. *Identify key performance indicators to measure.* These should have a direct link to customer needs and expectations. Typical performance indicators are quality, performance, and delivery.

3. *Identify the best-in-class companies.* For specific business functions, benchmarking might be limited to the same industry. For generic business functions, it is best to look outside one's own industry. Selecting companies requires knowledge of which firms are superior performers in the key areas. Such information can be obtained from published reports and articles, industry experts, trade magazines, professional associations, former employees, or customers and suppliers.

4. *Measure the performance of the best-in-class companies and compare the results to your own performance.* Such information might be found in published sources or might require site visits and in-depth interviews.

5. *Define and take actions to meet or exceed the best performance.* This usually requires changing organizational systems. Simply emulating the best is like shooting at a moving target—their processes will continually improve. Therefore, attempts should be made to exceed the performance of the best organizational systems.

Quality Improvement Process Steps

Process steps describe the interrelated tasks that lead to a potential improved outcome. These tasks include analyzing and responding to problems. Although some quality management specialists view their problem-solving processes as unique, the processes used by quality teams follow well-known team decisionmaking and problem-solving procedures. The typical problem-solving process followed by a management team has six steps:

1. Defining the problem, including identifying where to look for potential problems
2. Planning for solutions; collecting data
3. Translating processes into actions
4. Taking action

5. Evaluating actions and the desired outcomes for impact
6. Rediagnosing the problem and taking new actions as necessary

A well-known approach used by the Hospital Corporation of America, based on Deming's work, is labeled FOCUS-PDCA (Plan, Do, Check, Act) and encompasses nine steps;[13]

1. Find a process to improve
2. Organize a team that knows the process
3. Clarify current knowledge of the process
4. Understand the causes of process variation
5. Select the process improvement
6. Plan—improvement and data collection
7. Do—improvement, data collection, and data analysis
8. Check—data for process improvement, customer outcome, and lessons learned
9. Act—to hold the gain and continue improvement

This process flow is a variation of the well-known organizational development procedure that relies on four steps—diagnosis, planning, action, and evaluation—which are conducted in a continuous cycle. Consistent with quality management philosophy, collection of data and analysis of facts are relied on throughout the process.

Measurement Challenges

A critical point of quality management philosophy is that data and facts are used to assist in making the diagnosis, in establishing a plan for intervention, and in assembling the evidence that determines whether quality improvement has occurred. How data are collected can determine their accuracy and their use in monitoring the process of care. Computerized patient record systems are the most reliable automated data source; automated claims systems may be the least reliable. Combining automated and chart review data provides the best results in identifying quality of care—the NCQA calls this the hybrid methodology of data collection. Multiple data sources, as opposed to single data sources, are also more accurate in determining appropriate quality.

Value profiles for hospitals are based on data from outcome measures, costs, patient mix, severity, and processes of care to allow purchasers to select preferred sources of health care. As an example of value profiles, the Pennsylvania Health Care Cost Containment Council (*www.phc4.org*) has collected data that identify specific hospitals, physicians, and procedures, and their risk-adjusted outcomes for in-patient services.

Batalden and Nelson developed the Clinical Value Compass, which has four dimensions: (1) functional status, risk status, and well being; (2) costs; (3) satisfaction with health care and perceived benefit; and (4) clinical outcomes.[14] Figure 1–2 describes the Clinical Value Compass and gives an example of its use for hypertension.

In 1999, Bates showed that data collected at the point of care through an integrated information system could have great impact on the quality of care, including improved use of evidence-based medicine.[15] The costs of quality improvement in a health care organization can also be justified through appropriate data collection. For example, patient outcomes and satisfaction can be correlated with billing data, showing that quality improvement expenditures can produce tangible benefits. Expenditures for disease and population-management programs may markedly improve clinical outcomes, patient satisfaction, and provider satisfaction, while decreasing the cost of care.

Figure 1–2   Clinical Value Compass

1) Functional Health Status
- Physical
- Mental
- Social/Role
- Risk Status
- Perceived Well-being

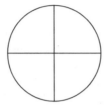

4) Biological Status (outcome)
- Mortality
- Morbidity

3) Satisfaction Against Need
- Health Care Delivery
- Perceived Health Benefit

2) Cost
- Direct Medical
- Indirect Social

Performance Patterns

Results of the interaction among patient, staff, and clinical and support processes produce patterns of critical results—biological outcomes, functional status and risk outcomes, patient perspectives of quality of care, and cost outcomes that combine to represent the value of care.

Clinical Value Compass

The Clinical Value Compass presents a balanced approach to measuring and displaying value in health care. It is a measurement designed for identifying and monitoring those key indicators of care that enable one to assess the quality of health care. The compass provides a framework for measuring changes in four major categories of health care value:

- Biological status
- Functional status
- Patient expectations and satisfaction
- Costs

While defining the broad categories of measures, the Clinical Value Compass leaves decisions regarding which specific measures are to be used for each indicator and each population to the various practice environments.

Quality management and improvement would be much less intimidating without the measurement challenges that arise at nearly every point in the quality improvement process. These challenges involve the availability and access of data, standardization, data quality, validity of

Figure 1–2   Clinical Value Compass (continued)

1) Functional Health Status
- Baseline Questionnaire

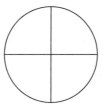

4) Biological Status
- Short Term:
  - Controlled Blood Pressure
  - Diet Compliance
  - Med Compliance
  - Ideal Body Weight
- Long Term:
  - Stroke
  - Left Ventricular
  - Hypertrophy
  - Coronary Artery Disease
  - Kidney Function

3) Satisfaction Against Need
- Physician (Provider)
- Nurse Visit
- Process of Care

2) Cost
- Physician Visits
- Nurse Visits
- ED Visits
- Hospitalizations
- Medications

data, reliability, the need for multiple streams of information, timeliness, and costs. Table 1–5 shows the comprehensive methodology used for collecting Health Plan Employer Data and Information Set (HEDIS) data for cervical cancer screening. It identifies the need for specific methodology, and the complexities of data collection, even with an excellent work tool.

1. *Availability and access.* Traditionally, quality improvement has involved a struggle between using data that are available and taking on the challenge of collecting new information that precisely answers the quality questions being asked. Thus, the literature contains much discussion about the usefulness of available administrative databases for addressing issues of quality of care.[16] The trade-off is the time and cost required to collect the precise data needed.

2. *Standardization.* Quality improvement has always involved comparing the processes and performance of one organization with another. The difficulty is that processes for data collection are rarely standardized across organizational boundaries. The lack of standardization can render comparisons meaningless (e.g., patient satisfaction numbers presented by different managed-care organizations). Discrepancies exist because instruments used to collect patients' perspectives and the ways in which data are collected do not match. To remedy the situation, standard methodologies for quality improvement studies are beginning to be adopted by health care organizations,

Table 1–5   HEDIS Methodology for Cervical Cancer Screening (CCS)

SUMMARY of CHANGES to HEDIS 2005

- Added LOINC to Table E7-A to identify cervical cancer screenings.
- Clarified Table E7-1/2 data elements for reporting.

DESCRIPTION

The percentage of women 18–64 years of age who received one or more Pap tests during the measurement year or the two years prior to the measurement year.

ELIGIBLE POPULATION

Product lines	Commercial, Medicaid (report each product line separately).
Ages	Women 21–64 years as of December 31 of the measurement year.
Continuous enrollment	*Commercial:* The measurement year and the two years prior to the measurement year.
	Medicaid: The measurement year.
Allowable gap	No more than one gap in enrollment of up to 45 days during each year of continuous enrollment. To determine continuous enrollment for a Medicaid beneficiary for whom enrollment is verified monthly, the member may not have more than a 1-month gap in coverage (i.e., a member whose coverage lapses for 2 months [60 days] is not considered continuously enrolled).
Anchor date	Enrolled as of December 31 of the measurement year.
Benefit	Medical.
Event/diagnosis	None.

ADMINISTRATIVE SPECIFICATION

Denominator	The eligible population.
Numerator	One or more Pap tests during the measurement year or the two years prior to the measurement year. A woman had a Pap test if a submitted claim/encounter contains any one of the following codes:

Table E7-A: Codes to Identify Cervical Cancer Screening

CPT Codes	LOINC	ICD-9-CM Codes	UB-92 Revenue Codes
88141-88145, 88147, 88148, 88150, 88152-88155, 88164-88167, 88174-88175	10524-7, 18500-9, 19765-7, 19766-5, 19764-0, 19762-4, 19774-9, 33717-0	91.46 *V Codes:* V76.2	923

Exclusion (*optional*):

Women who had a hysterectomy and who have no residual cervix and for whom the administrative data does not indicate that a Pap test was performed. The MCO should look for evidence of a hysterectomy as far back as possible in the member's history, through either administrative data or medical record review. The hysterectomy must have occurred by December 31 of the measurement year. The MCO may use any of the following codes in Table E7-B to identify allowable exclusions:

Table E7-B: Codes to Identify Exclusions for Cervical Cancer Screening

Description	CPT Codes	ICD-9-CM Codes
Surgical codes for hysterectomy	51925, 56308, 58150, 58152, 58200, 58210, 58240, 58260, 58262, 58263, 58267, 58270, 58275, 58280, 58285, 58290-58294, 58550, 58551, 58552-58554, 58951, 58953-58954, 59135, 59525	68.4-68.8

Table 1–5	Methodology for Cervical Cancer Screening (CCS) (continued)

HYBRID SPECIFICATION

Denominator   A systematic sample drawn from the eligible population for each product line. The MCO may reduce the sample size using the current year's administrative rate or the prior year's audited, product line-specific rate.
Note: For information on reducing the sample size, refer to the Guidelines for Calculations and Sampling.

Numerator   One or more Pap tests during the measurement year or the two years prior to the measurement year as documented through either administrative data or medical record review.

Administrative   Refer to the *Administrative Specification* above to identify positive numerator hits from the administrative data.

Medical record   Documentation in the medical record must include both of the following:
- a note indicating the date the test was performed, *and*
- the result or finding.

Exclusion (*optional*):

Refer to the *Administrative Specification* above for exclusion criteria. Exclusionary evidence in the medical record must include a note indicating a hysterectomy with no residual cervix. The hysterectomy must have occurred by December 31 of the measurement year. The MCO may use the descriptions of the codes listed in Table E7-B as synonyms for a hysterectomy with no residual cervix.

Note: The MCO should count toward this measure any cervical cancer screening methodology that includes the collection and microscopic analysis of cervical cells. The MCO may not count biopsies for this measure because they are used for diagnostic and therapeutic purposes only and are not valid for primary cervical cancer screening.

Data Elements for Reporting

An MCO that submits HEDIS data to NCQA must provide the following data elements:

Table E7-1/2: Data Elements for Cervical Cancer Screening

	Administrative	Hybrid
Measurement year	X	X
Data collection methodology (administrative or hybrid)	X	X
Sampling method used		X
Eligible population	X	X
Number of numerator events by administrative data in eligible population (before exclusions)		X
Current year's administrative rate (before exclusions)		X
Minimum required sample size (MRSS) or other sample size		X
Oversampling rate		X
Final sample size (FSS)		X
Number of numerator events by administrative data in FSS		X
Administrative rate on FSS		X
Number of original sample records excluded because of valid data errors		X
Number of records excluded because of contraindications identified through administrative data		X
Number of records excluded because of contraindications identified through medical record review		X
Number of employee/dependent medical records excluded		X
Records added from the oversample list		X
Denominator		X
Numerator events by administrative data	X	X
Numerator events by medical records		X
Reported rate	X	X
Lower 95% confidence interval	X	X
Upper 95% confidence interval	X	X

Source: National Committee for Quality Assurance

accrediting bodies, and regulators. NCQA has even had certified audits of many of its HEDIS outcomes and Consumer Assessment for Health Plan Summary (CAPHS) outcomes.

3. *Data quality.* At every level of quality management attention—individual, team, unit, organization, or community—data quality is critical. The level of confidence inspired by the data that are examined for quality improvement purposes depends on the care with which data are collected and presented to the organization. Missing or misrepresented data can easily skew the results of the survey or performance review.

4. *Validity.* Much has been made about the problem of validity in quality management. A key question to ask is, "Do the measures selected to indicate the presence or absence of quality actually represent quality in the patient care experience?" Overall, the validity of the indicators and monitors selected needs to be examined to determine if it really represents quality outcomes. Mortality—an example of a crude measure—is sometimes considered an indicator of quality. Unexpected mortality brings the quality of patient care into question. Unfortunately, the indicator is not prevalent enough to be meaningful, and many variables besides clinical transactions affect outcome. Thus, the validity of mortality as a quality measure may not be accurate without further investigation.

5. *Reliability.* Quality indicators must yield the same results when measured repeatedly. In other words, measurement indicators and data collection techniques must be stable enough to justify the use of the collected information in making a judgment about quality. The same measurement process using the same data should produce the same results.

6. *Multiple streams of data.* It is tempting to use a limited number of indicators to judge the quality of patient care delivered in an organization. But the conceptual and theoretical leaders of the field, such as Donabedian,[2] state that understanding quality in all its richness requires information about structure, process of care, and outcomes. This requirement mandates multiple streams of data. Unfortunately, the more complex the data requirements, the more difficult the quality management task becomes.

7. *Timeliness.* A seemingly less complex challenge—measurement timeliness—is in fact one of the most difficult challenges to address. Quality data are needed when the quality teams are ready to act, when regulators are ready to review them, and when medical and administrative leaders are making strategic decisions about quality in the organization's future. Delivery of the data later is unacceptable but common. Most administrative data sets are more than 30 days old. The advent of electronic data interchange will help streamline the timeline of administrative data. The most up-to-date administrative data usually come from the pharmacy, where the data are usually processed the same day that they are obtained and thus made available for data collection.

8. *Costs.* A great challenge to quality measurements is the cost of addressing the weaknesses in existing quality improvement efforts, especially in data systems.[17] To improve the scope and depth of quality data, organizations have invested substantially in information system hardware and software. However, even more must be invested in data capability to satisfy the critics of quality measurement. A conflict arises when clinicians believe that the enormous expense of creating and maintaining data systems undercuts the availability of resources for clinical care. The more effort that is made to address quality management challenges, such as obtaining multiple streams of data, the more the cost question comes into play. It is possible to use the old streams-of-quality data that are valid and reliable, standardized across organizations, and available when needed, but the

cost to the organizations and to the health system is quite high. For example, collecting clinical data from a chart review costs $80 to $100 per hour. This cost only covers extracting the data from the chart and importing them into the information system. The programming for the information system can cost an additional $150 to $300 per hour, depending on the interfaces and software builds needed to allow the data to be used in the quality improvement program.

9. *Risk adjustment.* Another great challenge to measurement is risk adjustment, which is a method of comparing illness among individuals or populations with the same primary diagnosis. The mix of patients with regard to health status, demographics, illnesses, and severity of illness can vary from one health care organization to another. Unless these differences are taken into account, comparing one organization to another may be unfair. Co-morbidities can affect the primary diagnosis and increase or decrease the risk or severity.

Controversy exists in the use of risk adjustment. Iezzoni concluded that severity-adjusted mortality rates do not explain quality differences across hospital systems and expressed concern about the use of the assessment mechanisms in determining the quality of hospital care.[18] To adjust appropriately for risk, a strict definition of each specific outcome is required. Indicator data need to be selected wisely and collected carefully, and they must be as free from potential bias as possible. Appropriate multivariate model-building procedures should be used, and the final score should be evaluated for reliability and validity.

Understanding risk adjustment is vital because risk adjustment is becoming an important financing mechanism for health care. Risk adjustment is now being applied to populations in several governmental and commercial plans; examples include state and federal programs that use ambulatory care groups, risk adjuster categories, or diagnostic-related groups. In a simple form of risk adjustment, some employers are increasing the premium sharing to employees who report unhealthy habits, such as smoking.

The Veterans Administration system has become a leader in severity adjustment and outcomes improvement. In Veterans Administration hospitals, Khuri and Daley developed a multivariable risk-adjustment model that predicted 30-day morbidity and mortality rates for patients undergoing 123 specific types of surgery.[19] The buy-in of the surgeons, consistent clinical definitions, dedicated data collection resources, a uniform informatics system, and the support of senior management were the key successes of this program.

Another type of comparison that has been used for many years is the Episode of Care (EOC). Clinical, financial, resource-use, and administrative data are collected for a defined period about all cases of a single intervention or aspect of care, such as kidney dialysis or myocardial infarction. Specific EOCs from various departments or institutions can then be compared, provided that the results are adjusted for diagnosis, case mix, comprehensiveness of data collection, and clinical flexibility. Table 1–6 presents a short narrative about the risk adjustment methodology used by the state of Maryland for its Medicaid Managed Care population. The narrative shows that risk adjustment is a complex process that involves many factors.

With all of these measurement challenges, a major issue that emerges is which data to use and how to use them. Making summative judgments about quality—poor, good, outstanding—requires great confidence that the previously mentioned challenges have been met. If concern about the data is substantial, the information can be used to induce a dialogue about the state of quality—a formative discussion that avoids summative judgments (which are precluded by the lack of confidence in the data). Healthy skepticism should always be maintained in judging the validity of the data, but even more so in judging how the data are interpreted and converted to information.

Table 1–6   Payment Methodology and Risk Adjustment Model for Medicaid (State of Maryland)

A Medicaid managed care plan pays each participating managed care organization (MCO) demographic and risk-adjusted capitation for waiver-eligible Medicaid recipients. Supplemental or separate rates are paid by the Medicaid managed care plan to each MCO for (1) maternity/delivery care, (2) persons living with HIV/AIDS, and (3) pregnant women eligible under the Sixth Omnibus Reconciliation Act (SOBRA).

Payment Methodology

The Medicaid managed care plan sets capitation rates for two broad eligibility categories of enrollees: families and children, and persons with disabilities. These rates are calculated by the Medicaid managed care plan by trending forward audited MCO medical and administrative costs for a base year. For new Medicaid recipients and those with less than 6 months of eligibility during the base year, the Medicaid managed care plan sets specific rates based on demographic factors. For those Medicaid recipients with at least 6 months of eligibility during the base year, the Medicaid managed care plan uses the Ambulatory Care Group (ACG) case-mix methodology developed by Johns Hopkins to assign recipients into risk-adjusted categories. In summary, the Medicaid managed care plan establishes two core rate structures for each eligibility group—temporary aid to needy families (TANF) and supplemental security income (SSI)—demographic rates and risk-adjusted rates.

Risk Adjustment

1. Demographic Factors
   The Medicaid managed care plan uses three demographic factors—age, gender, and location—to adjust its capitation rates for new Medicaid recipients. The age groupings are (1) under 1, (2) age 1–5, (3) age 6–14, (4) age 15–20, (5) age 21–44, and (6) over 45. These groupings are also adjusted for gender (male/female) as well as location (city/rest of state).
2. Risk-Adjusted Factors
   The Medicaid managed care plan uses the ACG system to assign each enrollee into one of the ACG categories. Each ACG category is designed to represent individuals with similar morbidity and/or expectations for health care resource consumption. In recognition of the administrative complexities of making payments to MCOs based on ACGs, the Medicaid managed care plan consolidates the 80+ ACGs into 18 risk-adjusted categories (RACs). The RACs are divided based on the two broad eligibility categories: (1) RACs 1–9 for families and children and (2) RACs 10–18 for persons with disabilities. In general, enrollees assigned to higher RACs are expected to consume more health care resources.[20]

Information Systems Support: Indicators and Monitors

What is it that quality managers must monitor? Information must support every aspect of quality improvement activity. For example, does the trauma-center team monitor only mortalities? Or is the team also interested in how quickly the pre-hospital emergency services system delivers the injured patient to the hospital (e.g., within the "golden hour")? Many medical and administrative leaders track overall results but not the details of their processes, an error highlighted by one commentator:

> Managers spend too much time looking at published results and not enough looking at what drives those results. Most chairmen know their company's overall return on sales. Surprisingly few know what percentage of their products are delivered on time or what the age-profile of their machinery is. Such figures are often not even collected. That is rather as if a tennis player watched the scoreboard, but not the ball."[21]

Information systems are covered in Chapter 5, and only a few concerns—such as purposes, sample measures, and applications—are addressed here. The information system is required to support the quality effort in all aspects of its operation, meeting the needs defined by the Institute of Medicine:[22] supporting patient care and efforts to improve quality, supporting clinical and health services research (and evidence-based medicine), and protecting patient confidentiality.

Indicators used in quality management vary by level and by organization. Some sample indicators are:

- In-hospital mortality
- Hospital-acquired complications
- Severity-adjusted outcomes (e.g., surgical, obstetrical)
- Patient satisfaction
- Attempted suicide
- Provider availability and accessibility
- Delay in care
- Patient-initiated complaints
- Transfer to a higher level of care

The National Quality Forum has compiled a list of serious reportable events that can be used as sentinel events for various health care organizations (see Table 1–7).

Although a single indicator is usually not rich enough to use as a stand-alone tool for assessing quality, a set of indicators begins to provide confidence for judgment. For example, a set of indicators for examining the outcomes of pregnancy and newborns is shown in Table 1–8 (page 29). The use of this set may give an organization a more complete look at the quality of care being delivered to its pregnant women and may reveal potential quality issues.

To support organization-wide quality improvement work, information systems would ideally be expected to:

- Use computer-based patient records
- Have computerized order entry
- Include clinical services tracking
- Include ambulatory care services tracking
- Include nursing services
- Support clinical decisionmaking systems
- Include computer-assisted medical instrumentation

Although great gains are being made in system design, an information system's usefulness to the quality endeavor should have the following characteristics:

- Information—not data
- Relevant
- Sensitive
- Unbiased
- Comprehensive
- Timely
- Action-oriented

Table 1–7   Serious Reportable Events

Event	Additional Specifications
1. SURGICAL EVENTS	
A. Surgery performed on the wrong body part	Defined as any surgery performed on a body part that is not consistent with the documented informed consent for that patient.
	Excludes emergent situations that occur in the course of surgery and/or whose exigency precludes obtaining informed consent.
	Surgery includes endoscopies and other invasive procedures.
B. Surgery performed on the wrong patient	Defined as any surgery on a patient that is not consistent with the documented informed consent for that patient.
	Surgery includes endoscopies and other invasive procedures.
C. Wrong surgical procedure performed on a patient.	Defined as any procedure performed on a patient that is not consistent with the documented informed consent for that patient.
	Excludes emergency situations that occur in the course of surgery and/or whose exigency precludes obtaining informed consent.
	Surgery includes endoscopies and other invasive procedures.
D. Retention of a foreign object in a patient after surgery or other procedure	Excludes objects intentionally implanted as part of a planned intervention, and objects present prior to surgery that were intentionally retained.
E. Intraoperative or immediately post-operative death in an ASA Class I patient	Includes all ASA Class I patient deaths in situations where anesthesia was administered; the planned surgical procedure may or may not have been carried out.
	Immediately post-operative means within 24 hours after induction of anesthesia (if surgery not completed), surgery, or other invasive procedure was completed.
2. PRODUCT OR DEVICE EVENTS	
A. Patient death or serious disability associated with the use of contaminated drugs, devices, or biologics provided by the health care facility	Includes generally contaminants in drugs, devices, or biologics regardless of the source of contamination and/or product.
B. Patient death or serious disability associated with the use or function of a device in patient care in which the device is used or functions other than as intended	Includes, but is not limited to, catheters, drains, and other specialized tubes, infusion pumps, and ventilators.
C. Patient death or serious disability associated with intravascular air embolism that occurs while being cared for in a health care facility	Excludes deaths associated with neurosurgical procedures known to present a high risk of intravascular air embolism.
3. PATIENT PROTECTION EVENTS	
A. Infant discharged to the wrong person	

Table 1–7   Serious Reportable Events (continued)

Event	Additional Specifications
B. Patient death or serious disability associated with patient elopement (disappearance) for more than four hours	Excludes events involving competent adults.
C. Patient suicide, or attempted suicide resulting in serious disability, while being cared for in a health care facility	Defined as events that result from patient actions after admission to a health care facility. Excludes deaths resulting from self-inflicted injuries that were the reason for admission to the health care facility.
4. CARE MANAGEMENT EVENTS	
A. Patient death or serious disability associated with a medication error (e.g., errors involving the wrong preparation or wrong route of administration)	Excludes reasonable differences in clinical judgment on drug selection and dose.
B. Patient death or serious disability associated with a hemolytic reaction due to the administration of ABO-incompatible blood or blood products	
C. Maternal death or serious disability associated with labor or delivery in a low-risk pregnancy while being cared for in a health care facility	Includes events that occur within 42 days post-delivery. Excludes deaths from pulmonary or amniotic fluid embolism, acute fatty liver or pregnancy or cardiomyopathy.
D. Patient death or serious disability associated with hypoglycemia, the onset of which occurs while the patient is being cared for in a health care facility.	
E. Death or serious disability (kernicterus) associated with failure to identify and treat hyperbilirubinemia in neonates	Hyperbilirubinemia is defined as bilirubin levels > 30 mg/dl. *Neonates* refers to the first 28 days of life.
F. Stage 3 or 4 pressure ulcers acquired after admission to a health care facility	Excludes progression from Stage 2 to Stage 3 if Stage 2 was recognized upon admission.
G. Patient death or serious disability due to spinal manipulative therapy	
5. ENVIRONMENTAL EVENTS	
A. Patient death or serious disability associated with an electric shock while being cared for in a health care facility	Excludes events involving planned treatments such as electric countershock.

Table 1–7	Serious Reportable Events (continued)

Event	Additional Specifications

B. Any incident in which a line designated for oxygen or other gas to be delivered to a patient contains the wrong gas or is contaminated by toxic substances

C. Patient death or serious disability associated with a burn incurred from any source while being cared for in a health care facility

D. Patient death associated with a fall while being cared for in a health care facility

E. Patient death or serious disability associated with the use of restraints or bedrails while being cared for in a health care facility

6. CRIMINAL EVENTS

A. Any instance of care ordered by or provided by someone impersonating a physician, nurse or pharmacist, or other licensed health care provider

B. Abduction of a patient of any age

C. Sexual assault on a patient within or on the grounds of a health care facility

D. Death or significant injury of a patient or staff member resulting from a physical assault (i.e., battery) that occurs within or on the grounds of a health care facility

Source: National Quality Forum.

- Uniform (for comparative purposes)
- Performance targeted
- Cost-effective

Addressing these criteria is a lengthy process that is covered further in Chapter 5.

Methods and Tools

Quality of care can be assessed by any of several methods, including evaluations of patient reports, risk adjustment, assessments of health care settings, adherence to clinical practice guidelines, and examination of the degree to which information on quality tools and techniques have been disseminated to stakeholders. These methods emphasize looking at system variables, as it is now believed that system design problems are responsible for more mistakes and suboptimal outcomes than are errors by individuals. Whether analyzing systems or individual performance, quality managers need data, facts, and a scientific process to guide the work.

Quality Management Tools.
The eight most common tools of quality management are the problem-solving cycle, affinity diagrams, cause-and-effect (fish bone) diagrams, pareto diagrams, histograms, bar charts, scatter diagrams, and statistical control charts. The tools are explained below in the context of one hospital's

Table 1-8   Macro-Indicators for the Outcome of Pregnancy, Newborn Summary by Month

	Total	May '02	Apr '02	Mar '02	Feb '02	Jan '02	Dec '01	Nov '01	Oct '01	Sep '01	Aug '01	Jul '01	Jun '01
Number of Newborns													
Newborns													
Deliveries													
Average Gestational Age													
Newborns													
Count of Newborns by Gestational Age													
28 Weeks or Fewer													
29-34 Weeks													
35+ Weeks													
Infant Average Weight in Grams by Gestational Age													
28 Weeks or Fewer													
29-34 Weeks													
35+ Weeks													
Average Weight in Grams													
Count of Low Birthweight Babies													
Birthweight < 1500 grams													
1500–2500 grams													
2500+ grams													
Low Birthweight % of total delivered													
Birthweight < 1500 grams													
1500–2500 grams													
2500+ grams													

efforts to improve the quality of its patient discharge process, which is a troublesome event for many hospitals.

1. *The problem-solving cycle.* The tools of continuous quality improvement are used as part of an ongoing problem-solving cycle. Although many steps have been offered by adherents to the process, such as Deming,[4] Crosby,[5] and Juran,[3] the procedures seem to follow a four-step process that is familiar to organizational development practitioners—diagnosis, planning, action, and evaluation (see Section 3.0). This process is also called the Shewart cycle, or PDCA cycle, which stands for Plan, Do, Check, and Act.

During the "planning" stage of the Shewart cycle, the areas needing quality improvement are identified. These can be high-cost, high-volume, high-risk areas, or areas in which outcome results are not as good as the organization would like. The "doing" part of the cycle involves developing indicators and monitors, thresholds and benchmarks, and the methodology for the study intervention. The "checking" portion of the cycle involves collecting data from the doing portion and then producing information from those data. The final stage of the cycle is determining from the information whether the intervention produced improved outcomes as reflected in the information. If the intervention did produce improved outcomes, it may be continued to determine whether improvement can be maintained; if it did not produce improved outcomes, a new intervention is tried, and the cycle begins anew. The tools of data analysis and presentation described below are used at one or more points in this problem-solving process.

2. *Affinity diagram.* The technique of story boarding grew out of the film and cartoon industry; Disney Studios perfected it to an art form. In planning and organizational work, story boarding is more properly called an affinity diagram. The process begins with brainstorming, in which every participant writes ideas on separate cards and mounts those cards on a large corkboard or similar display (the story board). During a discussion, the ideas are rearranged according to subject matter—hence the term *affinity diagram.*

As the participants discuss the ideas and rearrange them into clusters, they identify subject headings and, to help the continuous quality improvement (CQI) process, they may identify the groups as causes, symptoms, impacts, or side-effects of the problem. The affinity diagram that results from the brainstorming session is typically used at the beginning of the CQI process. If affinity diagramming occurs later in the process, when individuals or group members are identifying actions for addressing immediate problems, the diagram will most likely contain alternatives that the group members have identified as actions to take. Table 1–9 describes brainstorming, and Table 1–10 explains how affinity diagrams are used.

3. *Cause-and-effect (fish bone) diagram.* The cause and effect diagram can aid in preventing premature action. Often referred to as a fish bone, or Ishekawa, diagram, it can be used to enhance the quality improvement team's ability to map the full range of possible root contributors to the desired outcome. A fish bone diagram is a graphical presentation of relationships among the fundamental variables on which the group will focus when initiating improvement action. The diagram is used to expand the group's purview and to begin to generate some consensus on targets for action. The fish bone tool is described in Table 1–11 and illustrated in Figure 1–3.

4. *Pareto chart.* Once themes and clusters of potential causes of a lack of quality in an area of care have been noted, the factors contributing most to the problem need to be identified. Quality managers may assume that all causes contribute equally to poor quality, or that one or more causes are the leading ones, without inspecting the data. Pareto diagrams, often expressed as bar graphs, help

Table 1–9	Creating Great Ideas by Brainstorming

What does this method do?

Provides a way of creatively and efficiently generating a high volume of ideas on any topic by creating a process that is free of criticism and judgment

Why use this method?

Encourages open thinking and team work.

Involves all team members.

Allows team members to build on each other's creativity while maintaining a unified goal.

For clarity, state the question to be discussed and write it down.

How do you effectively use this method?

Allow everyone to offer ideas without criticism!

Write each idea down, to be visible to all team members.

Review the list of ideas for clarity and to discard duplicates.

Table 1–10	Gathering and Grouping Ideas in an Affinity Diagram

What does this method do?

Allows a team to organize and summarize ideas after a brainstorming session, to better understand the essence of a problem and to possibly reach breakthrough solutions.

Why use this method?

Encourages creativity by all team members at all phases of the process.

Encourages creative connectivity of ideas and issues.

Allows breakthrough solutions to emerge naturally (even on long-standing issues).

Encourages participant ownership of results.

How do you effectively use this method?

Phrase the issue under discussion in a clear and complete sentence.

Brainstorm at least 20 ideas and issues and record each on sticky notes.

Sort ideas into related groups of 5 to 10 ideas.

Create summary or header cards using the consensus for each group.

show the relative contribution of the various causes of the problem. Table 1–12 describes the use of pareto charts, and Figure 1–4 presents a pareto chart that was developed to help a provider group examine its late discharges from a hospital.

5. *Histogram.* The histogram can help elucidate the reasons for a variation by depicting the frequency of each value of the quantitative variable. For example, the first step in understanding the reasons for variation in hospital discharge times is to choose a sample time, perhaps a two-week period, and to count the number of patients who were discharged during each hour throughout that

Table 1–11	Using a Fish Bone Diagram to Find and Cure Causes, Not Symptoms

What does this method do?

Allows a team to identify, explore, and graphically display in detail all of the possible root causes related to a problem or condition.

Why use this method?

Enables a team to focus on the content of the problem, not on the history of the problem or differing personal interests of team members.

Encourages support for resulting solutions through consensus.

Focuses the team on causes, not symptoms.

How do you effectively use this method?

Select the better of the two standard formats.

Generate the causes needed to build a cause-and-effect diagram.

Construct the fish bone diagram.

Figure 1–3	Fish Bone Diagram Illustrating Late Discharge from a Hospital

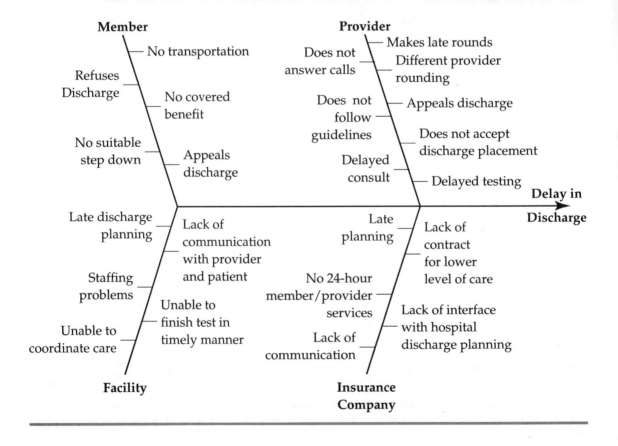

Table 1–12	Using a Pareto Chart to Focus on Key Problems

What does this method do?

Expends efforts on problems that offer the best possible improvement by showing their relative frequency or size in a descending bar graph.

Why use this method?

Helps a team to focus on causes that will have the greatest impact if solved.

Based on the pareto principle: 20% of the sources cause 80% of any problem.
Helps prevent "shifting the problem"; the "solution" removes some causes but worsens others.

How do you effectively use this method?

Decide which problem you want to know more about.

Categorize the causes or problems that will be monitored, compared, and ranked by brainstorming or with existing data.

Choose the most meaningful unit of measurement, such as frequency or cost.

Choose the time period for the study.

Collect the key data on each problem category either by "real time" or by reviewing historical data.

Compare the relative frequency or cost of each problem category.

List problem categories on the horizontal line and frequencies on the vertical line.

Interpret the results. Tallest bars indicate the largest contributors to the overall problem.

Figure 1–4	Pareto Chart to Examine Reasons for Delayed Discharge from a Hospital

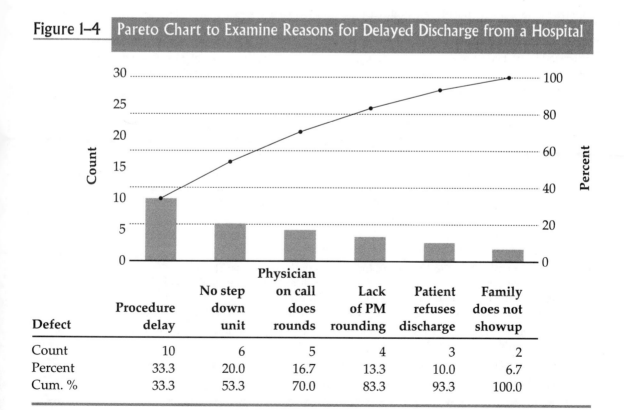

Defect	Procedure delay	No step down unit	Physician on call does rounds	Lack of PM rounding	Patient refuses discharge	Family does not showup
Count	10	6	5	4	3	2
Percent	33.3	20.0	16.7	13.3	10.0	6.7
Cum. %	33.3	53.3	70.0	83.3	93.3	100.0

period. The values can then be graphed on a histogram. The use of the histogram is explained in Table 1–13, and an example of a histogram is shown in Figure 1–5.

6. *Bar chart.* A bar chart is similar to a histogram, except that the variable of interest is not a quantitative measure, such as discharge time, but rather a categorical variable, such as a department within the hospital. Bar charts are commonly used to illustrate comparisons, such as the number of patients discharged before or after 11:00 a.m. for each of several hospital services, and may help identify departments that require further attention. As with histograms, bar charts are especially useful for diagnosis and evaluation. A bar chart that displays the number of laboratory tests performed by a physician group by month is shown in Figure 1–6.

Table 1–13	Using a Histogram to Achieve Process Centering, Spread, and Shape

What does this method do?

Aids in making decisions about a process or product that could be improved after examining the variation.

Why use this method?

Displays measurement data in bar graph format, distributed in categories.

Displays large amounts of data that are not easily interpreted in tabular form.

Shows the relative frequency of occurrence of the various data values.

Depicts the centering, variation, and shape of the data for easy interpretation.

Helps to indicate if the process has changed.

Displays the variation in the process quite easily.

How do you effectively use this method?

Gather and tabulate data on a process, product, or procedure (e.g., time, weight, size, frequency of occurrences, test scores, GPAs, pass/fail rates, number of days to complete a cycle, diameter of shafts built).

Calculate the rate of the data by subtracting the smallest number in the data set from the largest. Call this value R.

Decide about how many bars (or classes) to display in eventual histogram. Call this number K. This number should never be less than four and seldom exceeds 12. With 100 numbers, K = 7 generally works well. With 1,000 pieces of data, K = 11 works well.

Determine the fixed width of each class by dividing the range, R, by the number of classes, K. This value should be rounded to a "nice" number, generally a number ending in a zero. For example, 11.3 would not be a "nice" number, but 10 would. Call this number I, for interval width. The use of "nice" numbers avoids strange scales on the x-axis of the histogram.

Create a table of upper and lower class limits. Add the interval width to the first "nice" number less than the lowest value in the data set to determine the upper limit of the first class.

The first "nice" number becomes the lowest lower limit of the first class. The upper limit of the first class becomes the lower limit of the second class. Adding the interval width (I) to the lower limit of the second class determines the upper limit for the second class. Repeat this process until the largest upper limit exceeds the largest data piece. You should have approximate classes or categories in total.

Plot the frequency data on the histogram framework by drawing vertical bars for each class. The height of each bar represents the number.

Note the frequency of values between the lower and upper limits of that particular class.

Interpret the histogram for skew and clustering problems.

Figure 1–5   Histogram

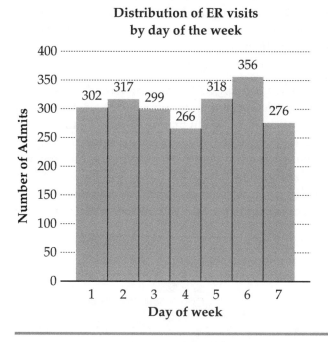

**Distribution of ER visits
by day of the week**

Figure 1–6   Bar Chart of Labtests by Month

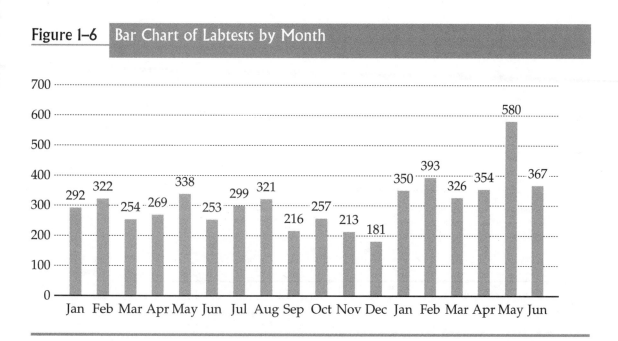

7. *Scatter diagram.* As noted, continuous quality improvement team members were charged with identifying those variables responsible for delaying a patient's discharge from the hospital. The possible causes of the delay included patient characteristics. One of the characteristics was the patients' length of stay in the hospital. The scatter diagram in Figure 1–7 shows the relationship between the length of stay and time of discharge and whether there is a pattern to this relationship; if so, the continuous quality improvement team would then investigate whether the pattern was controllable. Table 1–14 is a matrix explaining the use of a scatter diagram.

8. *Statistical control chart.* Processes typically have two kinds of variation; normal variation occurs under normal conditions, and abnormal variation occurs under unusual circumstances and can often be traced to a cause. A statistical control chart is a graph that represents continuous application of a particular statistical decision rule, to distinguish between normal and abnormal variations. Statistical control charts have been widely used to control quality in the management process. The use of a statistical control chart is explained in Table 1–15. Figure 1–8 shows a statistical control chart for the number of visits per day for a provider organization, covering each day during October of 2001. The UCL is the upper control limit, the LCL is the lower control limit, and the PCL is the process control limit.

Figure 1–7   Scatter Diagram Showing Correlation Between Length of Stay and Day of Admission

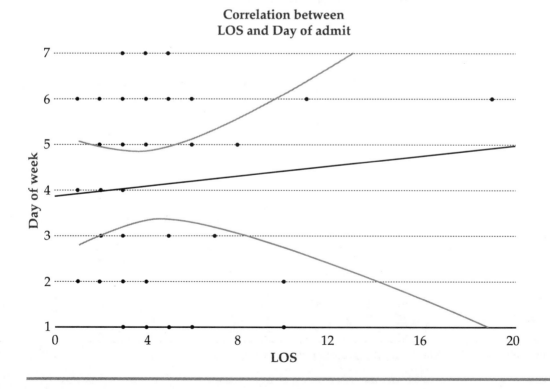

Table 1-14   Using a Scatter Diagram to Measure Relationships Between Variables

What does this method do?

Analyzes and identifies the possible relationship between the changes observed in two different measurements.

Why use this method?

Provides the data to confirm a hypothesis.

Depicts both visual and statistical means to test the strength of a potential relationship.

Provides a good follow-up to a cause-and-effect diagram to determine if more than a consensus connection exists between causes and the effect.

How do you effectively use this method?

Collect the data (50–100 paired samples of related data) and construct a data sheet.

Draw the x-axis and the y-axis, and plot points corresponding to these measures for each observation.

Interpret the data to determine if any pattern or trend emerges, noting positive or negative correlation.

Table 1-15   Using Control Charts to Recognize Sources of Variation

What does this method do?

Provides a comprehensive means to monitor, control, and improve process performance over time by studying variation and its source.

Why use this method?

Focuses attention on detecting and monitoring process variation and its source.

Distinguishes special from common causes of variation, as a guide to local or management action.

Serves as a tool for ongoing control of a process.

Provides a common language for discussing process performance.

How do you effectively use this method?

Identify the process to be charted.

Determine the sampling method and plan.

Initiate data collection:
    Run the process untouched, and gather sampled data.
    Calculate the appropriate statistics.
    Calculate the control limits.
    Construct the control charts.

Interpret the data:
    If any points fall outside the control limits, check for special causes of variation.
    If no points are outside the control limits, check for special causes of variation.
    If no points are outside the control limits, examine the data for non-random patterns.

Figure 1–8   Statistical Process Control Charts of Visits Per Day for a Physician Group

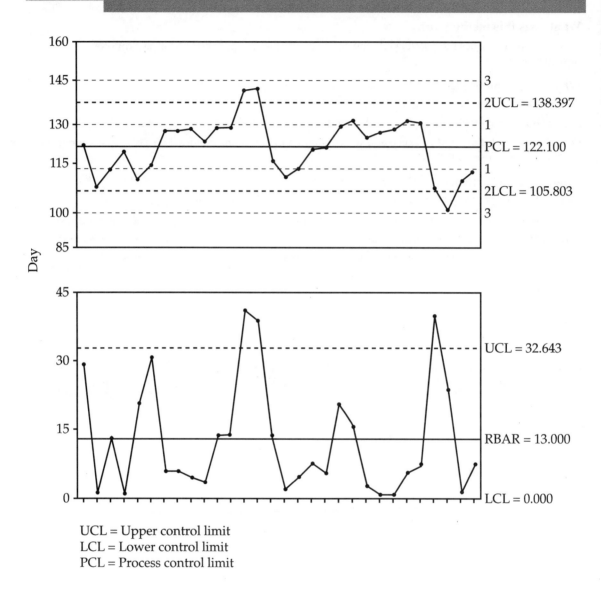

UCL = Upper control limit
LCL = Lower control limit
PCL = Process control limit

9. *Flow chart.* This chart allows the identification of the alignment of processes that need to be followed in the quality improvement project. It identifies the beginning and end of the process and how one part of the process is dependent on another. Table 1–16 is a matrix for the use of flow charts and Figure 1–9 is an example of a short generic flow chart.

Quality Improvement Methods.

Six important methods used in quality improvement are generic screens, surveys and feedback loops, practice guidelines, provider profiles, credentialing, and peer review. Each method may require the use of some of the data tools discussed in the previous section.

| Table 1–16 | Using a Flow Chart to Picture the Process |

What does this method do?

Allows a team to identify the actual flow or sequence of events in a process that any product or service follows.

Why use this method?

Shows unexpected complexity, problem areas, redundancy, and unnecessary loops, and reveals areas where simplification and standardization may be possible.

Compares and contrasts the actual versus the ideal flow of a process, to identify improvement opportunities.

Allows a team to come to an agreement on the steps of the process and to examine which activities may impact the process performance.

Identifies locations where additional data can be collected and researched.

Serves as a training aid for understanding and completing the process.

How do you effectively use this method?

Identify the boundaries of the process. Clearly define where the process in discussion begins and ends.

Team members should agree on the level of detail they must show on the flow chart, to clearly understand the process and identify problem areas.

1. *Generic screens.* Generic screens involve the routine monitoring of various processes in a health care system and have been in place for many years. The JCAHO has used them when reviewing hospitals, and several other organizations have used them to monitor the general quality of health care. In many cases, generic screens are "hand-me-downs" from previous quality assurance programs.

Generic screens are useful when they are triggered by sentinel events; that is, if the event is a one-time occurrence, the screen needs to be investigated. Some examples of sentinel events are:

- Maternal death during delivery
- Serious suicide attempt
- A lawsuit involving the health care organization or practitioner
- Major reaction to a prescription medication or blood transfusion
- Surgery performed on the wrong patient or the wrong site; the wrong surgical procedure performed
- Unexplained in-patient death

In other instances, the value of generic screens for improving performance does not justify the effort of collecting the data on them. Generic screens that are not triggered by sentinel events are useful if tracked by a specific methodology, such as statistical process control. The methodology should identify the need for an intervention when normal variation no longer explains the variation in the generic screen being monitored. These types of generic screens are changed frequently—perhaps quarterly—in the organization. A list of generic screens can be obtained from JCAHO and the American Accreditation Healthcare Commission/URAC. These screens can be used to monitor the processes and outcomes of care in health care organizations.

Figure 1–9   Flow Chart for Admission

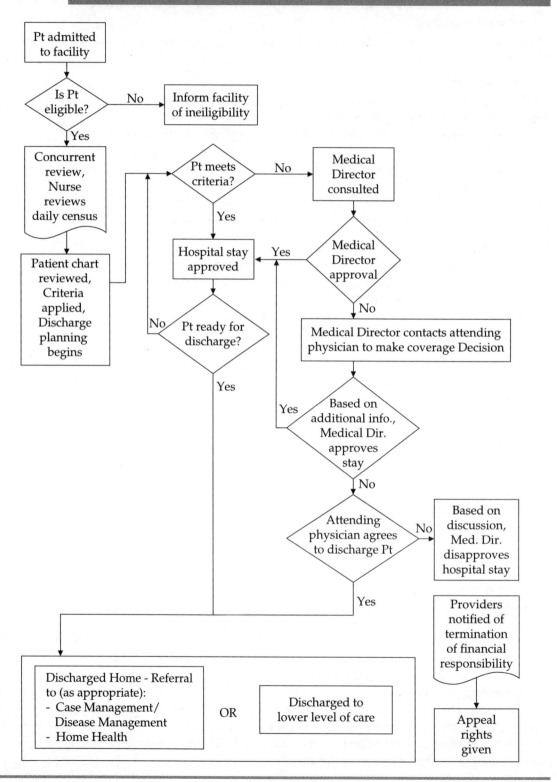

Pt = patient

2. *Surveys and feedback loops.* Surveys of patients and providers are commonly used in quality improvement, and can include a range of related methods, from mail surveys, to in-hospital surveys, to complaint letters and comments, to telephone surveys, to focus groups. Surveys are used to identify structure, process, and outcomes issues in the delivery of health care. They can identify the general impressions of a population or can collect detailed information about specific outcomes and delivery-of-care experiences. The typical order in designing and implementing a survey includes goal setting, method selection, instrument design, data collection, data processing, interpretation, and feedback. The objectives and expectations of the survey are critical to the interpretation of the survey results and to the probable use of the results.

The term "survey" is used in quality management to denote several different types of data collection and feedback strategies. The JCAHO conducts "surveys" of health care organizations to determine their accreditation-worthiness. The Malcolm Baldrige Quality Award is based on a "survey" that examines several aspects of organizational activity (see section 2.0.7). The notion underlying the survey is that high-quality organizations deliver high-quality care to patients. The surveys examine structure, and they ask for information about clinical processes and for reports on outcomes that demonstrate continued improvement of performance. These "organizational surveys" are widely used and are viewed as a primary tool for assessing current quality levels and for documenting improvement progress.

At another "level," surveys are administered to individuals—patients, employees, and purchasing customers—to determine what these stakeholders "individually" think of the quality of the care provided. Most surveys ask patients to address three elements of care: the technical aspects of care (i.e., the quality of diagnosis and therapeutic follow-up); the interpersonal aspects of care (i.e., friendliness, sensitivity, and helpfulness); and the amenities of care (i.e., the quality of support services, such as meals or the cleanliness of the patient's room). During early administrations of patient surveys, many clinicians objected that patients used clouded judgment that was influenced by nonessential amenities when they rated the clinicians' technical skills. But more recent research shows that patients rate the clinicians' experience in a holistic way, integrating technical, interpersonal, and amenities assessments into a global judgment.[23]

Patient surveys are common in hospitals, managed care plans, and clinical practices. Once dismissed as "mere collectors of amenities ratings," patient surveys are now regarded with much more respect and are viewed as one of the multiple streams of data needed to make a judgment about quality; however, their design and use continue to be challenging for the organizations administering the survey.

Designing and conducting a survey is a much more complex process than is often realized, and many surveys yield so much variation that the responses are meaningless. Survey data are affected by the construction and wording of the instruments, the sample size, the method of collection, the expectations of the patients, the type of patient, and the point of care at which patients are surveyed. Meeting these methodological challenges is critical to obtaining valid, reliable, and useful survey data. Unfortunately, even some simple solutions, such as using standardized, well-tested instruments, are ignored. NCQA produces one of the most standardized patient surveys, which is known as the Consumer and Patient Health Survey (CAPHS). It is used by many managed care organizations, and its results are used to compare patient satisfaction at one managed care organization with another.

Many organizations now have complaint systems that allow and encourage patients to feed complaints and concerns back to administrative and medical leaders. These complaint systems are used in tandem with surveys, or in some cases as separate feedback systems. The methods by which patients lodge complaints and grievances are now recognized by clinicians and policymakers as an important feedback mechanism. Medicare and Medicaid have made these feedback processes a strong part of their quality improvement programs, expecting that patterns of complaints will be addressed in the quality management programs of the health care organization. Ideally, the complaint process should be user-friendly, result in a quick response, and be seen as a tool for quality rather than a disciplinary tool. Table 1–17 presents a tool for recording grievances from a health care organization (complaints and appeals can be recorded in similar fashion), on which pertinent data for the follow-up of the appeal can be recorded.

3. *Practice guidelines.* Clinical practice guidelines are intended to improve health care by identifying optimal, evidence-based, medical practices.[24] They are usually developed to cover the normal routines of care. As they become more sophisticated, they cover more of the complicated processes of a disease. Such guidelines also address the issues of cost and quality in the practice of medicine, as well as patients' values and desires.

Technology assessment is also considered a form of guideline development, a best-practice approach synthesizing the results of literature reviews, consensus panel discussions, and expert opinions of new medical technologies. The National Guideline Clearing House at *www.guideline.gov* has collected over 961 guidelines that cover many clinical areas from various entities.

Guideline development is not uniform or easy. The most successful guidelines are based on valid information from credible sources, are applied in a receptive environment, and include incentives for following the guideline. Guidelines are often developed in a four-step process. First, the evidence for the intervention is analyzed to determine its effectiveness and the magnitude of its effect on particular outcomes. Second, the potential benefits and harms of the intervention are weighed. Third, if the benefits are determined to outweigh the harms, the costs of implementing the intervention are compared with the intervention's health effects. Finally, if resources are scarce, the priority for using the intervention is compared with that of other interventions. One method of developing a guideline is the Rand-modified Delphi method,[25] which brings clinical experts together to identify the steps in the appropriate treatment of a disease.

Grilli and Magrini reviewed 431 guidelines published by specialty societies in peer-reviewed journals[26] and found that only 22 met the following criteria: identifying stakeholders, specifying the search strategy for identifying published studies, and explicitly grading the strength of recommendations. These findings suggest that stricter criteria need to be followed in the development of guidelines. The British-based Cochrane Collaboration, the US Agency for Health Care Research and Quality, and NCQA all collect practice guidelines that meet strict methodological criteria.

Guidelines have been difficult to implement for various reasons. Many physicians see guidelines as "cookbook medicine," interfering with the physician-patient relationship. Others emphasize that evidence-based practice guidelines are not more reliable than the judgments of individual physicians. In any event, practice guidelines require considerable time and resources to develop and can become outdated with advances in medical care. Guidelines must be reviewed on a regular basis, or whenever a change occurs in the treatment or technology that addresses the clinical intervention.

Whether adhering to appropriate practice guidelines can decrease the amount of litigation in health care is still debated. The outcome probably depends on the nature of the guideline and the specifics of each case. However, the fact that a practice guideline was followed should help defend a case, assuming that care is documented and that the patient's condition was appropriate for applying the guideline. Computerized tracking and the use of an electronic medical record may help in the dissemination and use of guidelines.

Table 1–17   Grievance Recording Tool

Member Last Name	Member First Name	Plan Name	Member ID	

Address		City	State	Zip

Provider	PA	Claim	Type of Appeal	HBA Appeal #

Type of Service/Reason for Grievance	Member/Provider

Appeals Received	Month	Due Date	Acknowl Letter	DX Code

Claim #	Authorization #	Legal Rep

Grievance Level	Grievance Decision	Decision Date	Decision Letter

Upheld Reason	Overturn Reason

Medical Director Review and Sign Off

CEO Review and Sign Off

4. *Provider profiles.* If practice guidelines are developed by societies or specialty groups, the regional and national implementation of the guidelines by physicians should follow. Physician profiling could be considered the logical next step in monitoring guidelines. Profiles ("score cards" or "report cards") begin to identify how physicians practice. They may identify quality problems, utilization problems, or other potential areas of concern. Most of the profiles of individual physicians are obtained from claims-based data. Thus, the report card is only as good as the data that the physician submits. In addition, the profile may not have enough data to allow statistical analysis. The ability of the software to accommodate variations in data collection and classification may also be an issue.

Provider profiles are still in their infancy and can take many forms. Physician profiles have been aggregated to characterize an individual, a group practice, an academic section, an independent practice association (IPA), a managed care organization (MCO), a health maintenance organization (HMO), or other organizations that provide health care for patients. At the broadest levels, profiles will include indicators of quality, utilization, access, credentialing, complaints, and other areas thought to be important. An example of this aggregated level is the Health Plan Employer Data and Information Set (HEDIS) indicators for health plans. The individual health plan results are presented to the public in a report card so that potential clients can see how one health plan compares with another in the same geographic area. The NCQA's COMPASS report provides the same kind of comparison nationally for health plans.[27]

Figure 1–10 represents a simple physician profile that takes into consideration an individual physician's utilization patterns for bed days per 1,000 members, emergency department visits per 1,000 members, and referral rates per 1,000 members. The physician is given his or her ranking compared with rankings of physicians with the same specialty on the panel of the health care organization. The profile also includes a rolling quarterly average to enable the physician to determine if any interventions or changes in behavior have occurred. The profile is risk-adjusted for the population being served.

Although the potential usefulness of individual physician profiles should be recognized, five areas of concern should be noted when these profiles are examined: (1) the characteristics of the data used for the profile, (2) the clinical conditions being measured, (3) the accuracy of the data, (4) the latitude that the profiler has in altering or deleting data when the profile is developed, and (5) the time relevance of data collected. Even if all of these concerns are appropriately addressed, the physician should still carefully review the profile for accuracy. In addition, the profile should also reflect the severity of illness or risk adjustment for the patients whose data make up the profile. For example, sometimes an overall risk adjustment for the profile is compared with the average risk in the population that composes the physician's practice, or with the risk in a larger population group.

5. *Credentialing.* Credentialing is the process by which health organizations collect and review the education, training, and experience of professional caregivers. The documentation that is collected varies, but it often includes education and training, licensure, certifications, insurance, malpractice insurance, malpractice history, and other information deemed relevant for judging the suitability of the provider to deliver care. In general, the reliability of credentialing depends on whether the information supplied is complete, and whether it accurately represents the capability and experiences of the provider.

Figure 1–10 Physician Profile

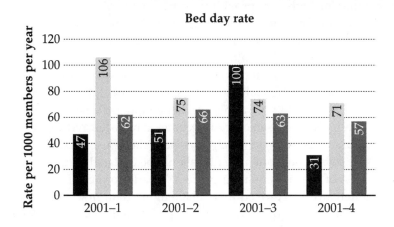

Bed day rate

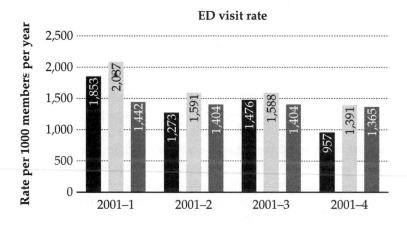

ED visit rate

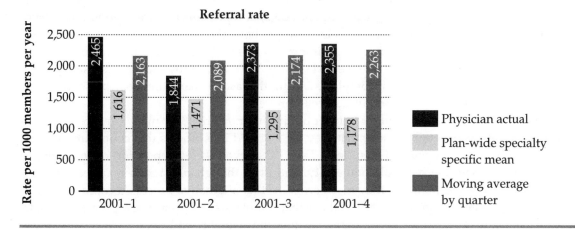

Referral rate

Quality managers often feel that highly capable providers (those vetted and credentialed by the organization) are likely to engage in high-quality clinical processes and procedures that lead to the desired patient outcomes. Screening for "sub-par" providers—a part of the old search for "bad apples"—was viewed as a way to raise quality levels by raising the minimum standards for recruiting and retaining providers. This screening was not viewed as a complex quality management task, but as a fundamental activity that was carried out almost automatically.

Unfortunately, successful credentialing is a difficult process. Collecting and analyzing the data is time-consuming and expensive, and the data often fall short of full disclosure. Initial credentialing can cost a health care organization $80 to $140 per applicant, depending on whether the credentialing program is conducted internally or is outsourced. Debates have occurred regarding whether credentialing should be a voluntary activity (in which physicians can refuse to participate), whether the data should be open to the public, how often the files should be updated, and, most importantly, who should pay for the cost of the credentialing process. To add to the difficulty, the technology of file creation and maintenance has proved more challenging than first anticipated. Nevertheless, credentialing remains a basic and required part of the quality management package. Most accrediting bodies have fairly uniform credentialing criteria for data collection and for the process that health care organizations must use to meet credentialing standards. Organizations like NCQA, JCAHO, AAAHC (Accreditation Association for Ambulatory Health Care), and URAC can be referenced for specific credentialing criteria.

6. *Peer review.* Peer review is the set of processes by which the appropriateness and adequacy of services is judged. It is best known as the mechanism by which Medicare reviews services for cost and quality. In more general terms, peer review connotes the review of clinical services by one's peers. Peer review organizations, now called quality improvement organizations (QIOs), review patient files, respond to complaints, learn from and correct errors, and work with individual physicians and facilities to prevent future errors. The concept that underlies peer review is that by examining the processes of care—the transactions between patients and providers—peers can render a second opinion on the appropriateness and adequacy of the services, answering the question, "Was the right thing done in the right way and at the right time?"

Peer review is intended to address the process of care by making a careful study of what actually happened during the patient's treatment episode(s); it represents a move beyond mere structural reviews that address such questions as, "Do we have the correct number of doctors and nurses, and are they qualified?" However, an important issue is the quality of the data provided to peer reviewers. In the early stages of the effort—in the 1970s and 1980s—reviewers using patient files frequently found them to be incomplete. During the last 10 years, immense pressure to improve documentation has arisen, and files have improved.

The peer review process is thought to be "punitive in orientation" by many physicians. However, peer reviewers generally believe that they are engaged in a process that contributes to continuing quality improvement of the system. The QIOs have taken the position of maintaining cordial relations with the medical community, and even though physicians may feel that the process is intrusive and punitive, they may recognize that alternative processes could be worse. Advocates for greater openness generally believe that complaints and peer review processes should be open to the public. At issue is the fundamental question of quality philosophy: Do we force quality improvement by public exposure and policing, or do we realize quality improvement by giving feedback, teaching, and providing opportunities for providers to continue giving care (armed with new knowledge)?

Outcomes Assessment

Although outcomes assessment is included as a separate method here, it is considered part of the whole quality effort. Outcomes assessment focuses on the third stage of Donabedian's model of structure, process, and outcome.[2] It involves careful study of the results of a patient's clinical intervention, which includes searching for impacts such as mortality and morbidity, functional status, and satisfaction. The assessment process asks, "What has happened to the patient?" The findings are compared with criteria and standards in the medical discipline to determine how the subject's care "measures up." Comparisons may be made by geographic area, patient type, provider organization, clinical intervention used, or individual provider. These comparisons typically require one or more of the following:

1. *Normative standards.* Developed as best practices in the field and by clinical and experimental trials, consensus conferences, and clinical models of high quality practice, these standards represent "the strived for."

2. *Benchmark standards.* Used with the collection of data from peer institutions and or consortia of institutions and departments, these standards represent the pooled professional judgment of people in the practice.

3. *Intra-organizational comparisons.* In these comparisons, outcomes for an organization are compared with previous and future data from that organization. The outcome measures are used to chart progress against the organization's own starting point, with the anticipation of reducing variability.

The methodology used in studying outcomes does not differ from normal scientific methodology. The data tools described previously are used in a driving effort to achieve scientific standards in research design and implementation (particularly in issues of measurement, such as reliability and validity). Many integrated approaches give attention to outcomes as well as their link to the interventions that are used in the process of care and service. In most outcomes studies, the outcome is considered significant if the intervention produces at least a 10% improvement in the outcome measure from the beginning to the end of the study.

Several regulatory and accrediting agencies' outcome measures are shown in Table 1–18. Also identified are the process objective and the selected outcome indicators. A more detailed discussion of outcomes assessment can be obtained from the Web sites of individual sponsoring organizations.

Another important outcomes assessment model is Healthy People 2010.[28] Table 1–19 identifies the health indicators and the proposed outcomes outlined in Healthy People 2010, which reflects the major public health concerns in the United States.

Integrated Approaches

Several approaches to quality management go beyond the tools and techniques of data tables, surveys, and other methods that have been discussed above. These approaches, including case and disease management, clinical pathways, evidence-based medicine, population health, Six Sigma, and demand management, all contribute to quality improvement knowledge and practice. They share the following characteristics:

- Focused on individuals and groups
- Not mutually exclusive
- Represent efforts to redesign systems

Table 1-18   Outcomes Evaluation Comparison

Sponsoring Organization	Initiative	Initiative Directed Towards	Process Objective	Selected Outcome Indicators and Criteria Measures
NCQA (National Committee for Quality Assurance)	HEDIS((Health Employer Data and Information Set)	Managed Care Organizations	Accreditation	14 primary measurement categories: childhood and adolescent immunizations, well visits for children and adolescents, prevention and ambulatory health, dental, asthma, heart disease, women's health (including breast and cervical cancer, Chlamydia), cholesterol management, hypertension, diabetes, behavioral health, and prenatal and postpartum care.
	CAHPS((Consumer Assessment for Health Plan Survey)	Managed care organizations	Data gathering, reporting and improvement/accreditation	2 primary measurement categories: access to treatment and services (primary care, specialty care, illness/injury), and experience with customer services (claims payment, customer service, complaint resolution).
JCAHO (Joint Commission on Accreditation of Healthcare Organizations)	ORYX®	Health care organizations and health professionals	Accreditation	4 initial core measurements for hospitals: acute myocardial infarction, heart failure, community-acquired pneumonia, and pregnancy and related conditions. Other core measurements being developed for each accreditation program. Examples: Long-term care to focus on adoption of MDS—Minimum Data Set; home care to focus on OASIS—Outcome and Assessment Information Set. Other non-core measures that can be selected from 100 performance measurement systems and thousands of performance measurements including (not inclusive): perioperative care, obstetrical care, CHF, respiratory care, ER care, rehabilitation care, immunizations, falls, antibiotic use.

Federal government				
	Healthy People 2010—US DHHS Office of Disease Prevention and Health Promotion	Health care organizations and health professionals	Data gathering, reporting, and best practices development	2 primary goals: increase quality and years of healthy life and eliminate health disparities. 10 leading health indicators: physical activity, obesity, tobacco use, substance abuse, responsible sexual behavior, mental health, injury and violence, environmental quality, immunization, and access to health care. 28 focus areas: access to quality health services; arthritis, osteoporosis, and chronic back conditions; cancer; chronic kidney disease; disability and secondary conditions; educational and community-based programs; environmental health; family planning; food safety; health communication; heart disease and stroke; HIV; immunization and infectious diseases; injury and violence prevention; maternal, infant and child health; medical product safety; mental health and mental disorders; nutrition and obesity; occupational safety and health; oral health; physical activity and fitness; public health infrastructure; respiratory disease; STDs; substance abuse; tobacco use; vision; and hearing.
	QISMC (Quality Improvement System for Managed Care)—US DHHS Centers for Medicare and Medicaid Services (CMS)	Health care organizations	Data gathering, reporting, best practices development, and regulatory oversight	Applicable to Medicare Advantage and Medicaid MCOs through BBA 1997. Organized in 4 primary domains (chapters): quality assessment and performance, enrollee rights, health service management, and delegation.
	Quality Interagency Coordination Task Force (QuIC)	Federal government agencies	Data gathering, reporting, and best practice development	Goal is to ensure that all federal agencies involved in purchasing, providing, studying, or regulating health care services are coordinated toward common goal of improving quality of care. Work groups are addressing specific projects within these 7 topic areas: patient and consumer information, improving quality measurement, developing the workforce, key opportunities for improving clinical quality (first 2 projects are diabetes and depression), improving information systems, reducing hazards in patient safety, and improving safety and quality through value-based purchasing.

Table 1–18 Outcomes Evaluation Comparison (continued)

Sponsoring Organization	Initiative	Initiative Directed Towards	Process Objective	Selected Outcome Indicators and Criteria Measures
	AHRQ Quality Indicators—US DHHS Agency for Healthcare Research and Quality (ARHQ)	Health care organizations and government agencies	Data gathering, reporting, and best practices development	Offshoot of HCUP, currently consisting of 3 quality indicator modules: prevention quality indicators (ambulatory care sensitive conditions), in-patient quality indicators (in-patient mortality for medical conditions; in-patient mortality for procedures, overuse, underuse or misuse of procedures; high volume/low mortality procedures) and patient safety indicators (Stanford Evidence-based Practice Center).
	CONQUEST (Computerized Needs-Oriented Quality Measurement Evaluation System)—US DHHS Agency for Healthcare Research and Quality (ARHQ)	Health care organizations, government agencies, and the general public	Data gathering, reporting, and best practices development	53 sets of quality performance measures to be assessed by consumers, purchasers, and health care plans/providers (e.g., HCUP, OASIS). Also includes a database containing information about 57 medical conditions.
URAC (American Accreditation Healthcare Commission)	Core accreditation standards	Health care organizations	Accreditation	The core standards are the foundation of URAC accreditation. These standards address several key organizational functions that are important for any health care organization, including organizational structure, staff qualifications, training and management, oversight of delegated activities, quality management, and consumer protection. The core standards must be met by all URAC-accredited entities (with the exception of Health Web Site) and serve as a prerequisite for the accreditation modules. Core accreditation can also be obtained by companies that provide services not addressed in URAC accreditation modules, such as pharmacy benefit management organizations, health education companies, and information technology (IT) and software firms.

	Disease management standards	Health care organizations	Accreditation	Standards in 4 accountability areas: scope and interventions offered, performance measures and methods, participant rights and responsibilities, population management methods, program design (including education and assessment).
	Health web site standards	Health care organizations	Accreditation	Standards in 4 accountability areas: scope and services offered, operations and processes, quality improvement, privacy and security, and delegation of responsibilities.
	Claims processing standards	Health care organizations	Accreditation	Key areas addressed include: timeliness of claims process, claims protocols, appeals processes, communications to claimants, staff training, and infrastructure.
NQF (National Forum for Health Care Quality Measurement and Reporting)	Develop nationally recognized quality standards	Across health care continuum	Data gathering, measurement, and reporting	Joint public/private organization to draft quality standards addressing: increased mortality and morbidity, failure to alleviate conditions that cause pain and disability, medical errors, over-treatment and under-treatment. US DHHS participating agency is Health Resources and Services Administration (HRSA).
FAACT (Foundation for Accountability)	FAACT/ONE	Health care organizations	Data gathering, reporting, and best practices development	Patient surveys in 5 areas: health care delivery (PCP), staying healthy (alcohol use), recovery and follow-up (major depressive disorder), living with chronic illness (asthma and arthritis), family needs during terminal illness.
CHAP (Community Health Accreditation Program)	Standards of excellence	Home and community health industry	Accreditation	4 primary framework focus areas having core and service-specific standards: structure and function (purpose, organization, administration, support of purpose), quality of services and products provided (accessibility, coordination, clinical policies and procedures, clinical records, quality improvement and client outcomes, infection control, and safety), resources (human, financial, physical), and long-term viability (planning, evaluation, risk management, marketing, accountability, expansion of knowledge, innovation). Received deeming authority for CMS (new HCFA) in May 1992.

| Table 1–19 | Healthy People 2010 Outcome Measures |

Indicator	Measurement for Outcome by Year 2010
Physical Activity	
1. Adolescent	85%
2. Adult	30%
Overweight/Obesity	
1. Children & adolescents	5%
2. Adults	15%
Tobacco Use	
1. Adolescent	16%
2. Adult	12%
Substance Abuse	
1. Drug-free adolescents	89%
2. Adult binge drinking	6%
3. Adult illicit drug use	2%
Responsible Sexual Behavior	
1. Adolescent	95%
2. Sexually active unmarried	95%
3. Partners using condoms	50%
Mental Health	
1. Adults treated for depression	50%
Injury and Violence	
1. Motor vehicle deaths	9.2 per 100,000 people
2. Homicides	3.0 per 100,000 people
Environmental Quality	
1. Exposed to ozone above EPA standard	0%
2. Exposed to environmental tobacco smoke	45%
Immunization	
1. DT&P, Polio, MNR, Hep B	80%
2. Influenza	90%
3. Pneumococcal	90%
Access to Care	
1. Persons < 65 years with health care coverage	100%
2. Persons of all ages with a specific source of ongoing primary care	96%
3. Females who received prenatal care in the first trimester	90%

Source: www.healthypeople.gov.

- Show a direct link between a process to an improved outcome based on current best practice and evidence-based medicine
- Involve patients in multiple areas of the health care organization
- Enhance the interaction between the patient and the care provider
- Fundamentally follow a continuous quality philosophy and practice in the clinical care of individuals and groups

Although these approaches are not new, they represent the current direction in continuing efforts to raise the level of care and to improve outcomes across institutions and systems. The basic concept of each approach and its contribution to quality management theory and practice is summarized below.

1. *Case and disease management.* The notion that quality increases if careful attention is paid to individuals and to groups of cases is not a breakthrough insight. But case and disease management must be considered part of the armamentarium used to meet the quality challenge, and the concept must be integrated with continuous quality improvement.

Case management has been defined as the centralization of planning, arranging, and following-up on a member's specific health services to manage utilization, effectiveness, and cost and quality, and to provide sustained or improved outcomes for the patient. Case management is a clinical system that strives to:

1. Coordinate the patient's care and monitor medical resource usage so that clinical and service interventions will have a positive effect and will result in sustained or improved outcomes.
2. Identify individual patients who may benefit from case management services (high cost, high risk, high volume; or patients with specific diseases or conditions that make them fragile).
3. Monitor the overuse, underuse, or misuse of services, and intervene to improve the outcome for the patient.
4. Identify barriers to care, and help to coordinate services or interventions that will have a positive effect on the patient's condition and will sustain or improve health outcomes.

A case manager is charged with the task of increasing the continuity of care and spurring collaboration among clinical and social service providers. In quality management philosophy, the case manager moves to alter the structure of care resources while maximizing the integration of clinical processes, with the expectation of enhanced outcomes.

Disease management is defined by the Disease Management Association of America as a system of coordinated health care interventions and communications for populations with conditions in which patient self-care efforts are significant.[29] The approach is an effort to maximize the quality of knowledge of disease states and treatment protocols using evidence-based medicine for specific patient groups, such as people with diabetes or congestive heart failure. The objective of disease management is to:

1. Support the provider of care and the patient-provider relationship.
2. Emphasize the prevention of exacerbations and complications, using evidence-based practice guidelines and patient-empowerment strategies.
3. Evaluate clinical, humanistic, and economic outcomes on an ongoing basis, with the goal of improving overall health.

The use of disease managers, information sharing, patient collaboration, and critical indicators are key components of disease management. Raising the level of focus and collaboration builds expertise and performance in clinicians and patients, and helps patients learn to self-manage their care at the highest level possible.

2. *Clinical pathways.* Clinical pathways have been defined as multidisciplinary plans of best clinical practice for specified patients with a single major diagnosis. These plans aid in coordinatng and delivering high-quality care, and they offer the potential of better outcomes for the patient. The use of clinical pathways is closely allied with the use of practice guidelines.

The principal objective of a clinical pathway is to reduce the variation in clinical processes that is thought to lead to differential outcomes; that is, to apply modern quality control methods. Although some variation is expected, because both patients and providers are individuals, carefully studying specific patient groups and following up by creating a common pathway for treating each patient group are thought to raise the quality of care by reducing activities and procedures that do not coincide with the group's consensus on best clinical process.

Typically, a committee of knowledgeable stakeholders—physicians, nurses, and ancillary staff—is convened to answer the question, "What must be done to the patient, and when must it be done?" All existing protocol steps and standing orders are reviewed, as are providers' differences in approach, use of resources, and expected outcomes. The committee charged with pathway development considers procedural schedules, targeted lengths of stay, selected outcome measures, and an analysis of the cost (i.e., potential gain or loss from the changes in procedures).

A contribution of the development of pathways is the studying and sharing of what was thought to be "common knowledge." The ensuing discussions have often revealed gaps, conflicts, and uncertainties. The use of clinical pathways provides shared learning about a common clinical process, redesign based on consensus, and care improvement and possible cost reduction. For example, a surgery pathway would use the following as outcome indicators: mortality rates, adverse occurrence rates, returns to surgery, infection rates, and other indicators identified by the stakeholders.

As noted for practice guidelines, clinical pathways can be developed for almost all procedures. The challenge is in communicating the pathways to staff, and in maintaining a constant upgrading of the process to reflect new procedural developments in each clinical area in the pathway. Using outdated pathways can do harm by locking the group into clinical processes that have been replaced by innovations; in such instances, variation may be reduced, but conformance to old standards may be counterproductive.

Some researchers believe that a group of clinical experts can use clinical pathways to decrease variation by developing practice guidelines and reviewing the practice of their peers. Others claim that variation will not appreciably decrease unless an electronic medical record is generated and appropriate documentation is gathered (i.e., unless a support capability is set up to drive the quality gain). Decreasing the variation and the rate of errors in medical practice has become a main area of concern for the federal government in its fight to improve outcomes for the population.

Competition, regulation, and professionalism—in addition to the use of clinical pathways—may help decrease practice variation. For example, a cardiac surgery program in New York found that regulation decreased risk-adjusted operative mortality rates by 41%.[30] Likewise, Maine physicians decreased variability by developing a culturally appropriate improvement program that included working together on common medical problems, involving respected local clinical leaders, and giving physicians direct feedback without public dissemination.[31] Although these programs are not the same as conscious clinical pathways processes, the spirit is similar.

3. *Evidence-based medicine.* Evidence-based medicine is a quality management concept that potentially affects all areas of medicine. The fundamental notion is that all medical care should be based on tested clinical trials with outcomes analysis; that is, medical knowledge should be put into practice constantly, and research should be used to test assumptions about care processes and outcomes. The call for this orientation is grounded in the belief that some medical care—perhaps too much—is based on intuition and untested logic, and that everything from therapeutic procedures, to equipment use and upgrades, to application of new drugs, is far "looser" (in terms of the connection between knowledge and practice) than would be expected from a science-based field. The quality questions are, "How much poor quality is from lack of *evidence* supporting the efficacy of a procedure?" and "How many practices are, in effect, based only on the "belief" that they make a positive contribution to patient care?"

The challenge in instituting evidence-based medicine is that the task is enormous. How can quality managers carefully examine all existing procedures and protocols, taking care to submit them to critical analysis and testing? The time and resource demands for such an endeavor are overwhelming. However, to disregard the task is to disregard the scientific basis of medicine and to ignore quality improvement's reliance on scrutiny of every aspect of clinical process. In some views, evidence-based medicine is the ultimate objective of quality improvement, wherein every aspect of clinical process is subjected to "scientific testing" of its contribution to patient care quality.[32]

4. *Population health.* Traditionally, quality management has been thought of as occurring within the boundaries of an organization (e.g., focused on individuals and groups within a hospital). Recently, quality managers have begun to think about managing the quality of care that is available to an entire community or population. This approach, defined as *population health*, requires attention to the full range of services, from preventive care, to primary care, to acute care, to long-term care. The quality objective is to examine structures and processes within a community or a defined population, to determine the opportunities for improvement. For example, improving the quality of care a patient receives in the operating room is possible, but a fundamental issue to consider is whether an opportunity exists to intervene in the health systems of a population to eliminate that patient's need for an operating-room visit in the future.

The literature on quality management is ripe with discussion of the uneven provision of services to populations and communities.[33] The Wennberg studies revealed that, in some communities, certain clinical procedures are far more common than in other communities.[34] The study raised important questions: "Why does this differential exist?" and, more importantly, "What is the nature of the quality problem?" and "Is the problem underprovision of services, or provision of services that are not needed (which raises the continued question of underuse, overuse, and misuse)?"

Managing the quality improvement process for a population is more complicated than that for smaller groups, but it requires the use of the same data-analysis tools and study protocols discussed previously. The added challenge is that the quality management effort crosses organizational boundaries and levels, thus necessitating the collaboration of hospitals, health care plans, physician practices, and long-term care providers. A particularly difficult issue is determining who takes the lead role: a health plan with an interest in protecting the health of its members, a health department as part of its community and public health effort, or a consortium of hospitals and other providers?

Along with the question of responsibility are issues of support for quality management activities (e.g., staffing, information systems, and resources). For example, quality managers have struggled to establish the information system capability within health care organizations. For quality management activities to be effective, this same capability must be present at the community and population levels.

Despite the challenges of population and community work, the benefits of this work should not be ignored. The opportunities to collaborate and provide continuity, to diffuse medical innovation, and to reduce variation within a community are clearly present. Healthy People 2010 is the population-based public health improvement program for the United States. Table 1–19 identifies the indicators and outcomes for Healthy People 2010. More information on this initiative can be found at *www.health.gov/healthypeople.gov.*

5. *Six Sigma.* Sigma is the 18th letter of the Greek alphabet and the symbol for standard deviation. The concept of Six Sigma was first introduced in the manufacturing area by General Electric and Motorola to improve quality, increase customer satisfaction, and save financial resources. It is now being utilized in service and health care organizations. The aim of Six Sigma is to reach a level

of quality that resides in the six standard deviations of average performance, giving an error rate of 0.0003% for the organization.

The objective of Six Sigma is to use data to identify quality problems, or potential quality problems, and areas for improvement. The Six Sigma approach concentrates on customer-driven measures and acceptable quality, and relies on data-driven process improvement. In this respect, it uses many of the tools previously identified in this chapter.

Six Sigma is generally instituted by practitioners trained in the use of the proper analytic tools to address quality problems. These practitioners are called "Six Sigma Black Belts." The Black Belts:

- Define the problem
- Measure the problem
- Analyze the data
- Improve the system
- Control and sustain the improvement

These actions are similar to the PDCA cycle that is used in other quality improvement programs.

For Six Sigma efforts to be successful, senior management must support them. These efforts cut across operational lines, use the most talented people in the organization, and move them into new areas. Six Sigma often brings culture shock to the organization, but it can produce a new culture of improvement. The Six Sigma concept is expected to become more popular in health care organizations over the next several years.

6. *Demand management.* Demand management is defined as the use of decision and self-management support systems to encourage and enable consumers to make appropriate use of medical care. The end result of demand management is the appropriate usage of health care resources, not decreased usage of health care resources. Demand has four components: morbidity, perceived need, patient preference, and non-health motives. Having morbidity or illness increases the patient's probability of seeking health care. Perceived need, which includes the knowledge of the risks a patient may have, the benefits of receiving care, the ability to assess the problem, and the confidence of the patient to care for the problem, may increase demand. Patient preference, which includes informed choice and shared decisionmaking about health care interventions, drives much of the demand for health care. Non-health motives include qualifying for sick leave or disability, and specific regulatory requirements for physical examinations or other interventions.

Present demand management programs concentrate on:

- Telephone contact by health care professionals (using decision support tools) for major interventions, such as surgery
- General communications for the use of the health care system, and care for minor health problems
- Population or individual care for the management of chronic disease
- Occupational or worksite prevention programs

Demand management usually enhances the services of the primary health care provider, and demand management programs empower the patient to use health care resources more prudently and can help to prevent the use of high-cost interventions. The overall savings for the health care system provided by this approach is still being debated.

Benefits and Outcomes of Quality Management

Organizations must have a mechanism that can identify potential quality problems at various levels—individual, team, unit, organization, and community—by examining structure, process, and outcome variables. In most cases, structural variables are in place and are of such quality that they do not greatly affect the outcome. However, process variables play an important role in the interventions that directly correlate with the outcome of care.

Outcomes can be evaluated from the standpoint of the patient, the payer, the regulator, or others. For example, a hip replacement procedure cannot be considered successful simply because the prosthesis has been positioned appropriately and the hip is functioning; the outcome must also be satisfactory to the patient.

In considering the benefits and outcomes of quality management, a key question to ask is, "What is to be gained from a quality management activity?" A comprehensive and effective quality improvement program should have an effect at each of five levels: individual, team, unit, organization, and community. The effects are generally thought of in three ways: patient care, financial gain, and individual and organizational development. The relationship among these effects is depicted in Figure 1–11.

As clinicians, most providers focus on patient care; that is, on the benefits that accrue to the patient. Reductions in variation in care, reductions in adverse consequences, and more efficient pathways to the desired clinical outcomes are real gains for the patient's system of care. This outcome

Figure 1–11   Tool for Monitoring the Effect of Quality Improvement

Benefits / Levels	Patient Care	Financial Gain	Individual and Organizational Development
Individual			
Team			
Unit			
Organization			
Community			

of quality improvement has been the first and foremost objective of quality management practitioners since Codman's work appeared nearly 100 years ago.[1]

A second outcome, financial gain, has perhaps received less attention than it should have. Crosby focused on the cost of poor quality and emphasized that poor quality not only affects patients negatively, but it also wastes resources that could be used to treat other patients.[5] Stressing the financial penalties for poor quality has gained the attention of administrative leaders who are debating whether to "invest" in the quality effort in health care. To see a return on investment is to convince managers that quality management has a business objective as well as a desirable benefit to patients.

For a quality study or program to be accepted by an organization, quality management professionals must present a cogent financial model with specific metrics and a specific return on investment. For example, the study could be identified in an issue paper that has specific areas of input. The paper should include:

- A short summary of the project and expected clinical outcome
- A roster of responsible parties, including the lead manager for the project and timelines for project implementation
- A comprehensive list of resources needed to make the project successful, and a description of other possible ways to conduct the project
- Recommendations to senior management that support the project

The third outcome, individual and organizational development, occurs as a by-product of examining structures, processes, and outcomes of care. Sharing data, opening new perspectives on procedures and care, and exposing outliers all help to educate clinical and administrative staff. Potential gains are: (1) the ability to use analytical procedures that require collection and analysis of data (a methodological development), and (2) the content that results from the analysis (which may give participants a richer sense of how their clinical structures and processes combine to produce the desired patient outcomes). The result is that both individuals and organizations are stronger because quality management is used.

Organizational Supports and Obstructions

Quality management can be either enhanced or undercut by the structural characteristics and behavioral dynamics of the organization. Outlined below are several leading issues in supporting and obstructing quality management.

Support Components

Although many issues are outside the immediate purview of clinical teams, several support components appear to be essential for a successful quality management effort: leadership, the presence of an advisory council, resources, information systems, training, incentives, and communication and feedback.

1. *Leadership.* Much literature on quality management emphasizes the importance of medical and administrative leadership.[35] The quality management leader provides the resources, personnel, and financial means to make the quality initiatives successful. The leader's contribution ranges from "kick off" speaker, to trainer, to liaison, to motivator. The leader's involvement in setting the strategic direction, in creating "celebration days," and in conducting periodic reviews of progress

is critical to the success of the effort. Also important are clinical leaders who support the quality initiatives and are willing to follow the clinical mandates of the quality program and bring along recruits. Importantly, employees at all levels often know immediately whether the new quality effort is "for show" or "for real."

2. *Advisory council.* The presence of a quality advisory council announces several points, such as many "hands" are needed to make this initiative work; this is an open and participative process; employees at all levels are welcomed and encouraged to join the effort; and the council can move the effort further faster.

3. *Resources.* Although Crosby put forth the notion that "quality is free",[5] the effort to initiate and sustain improvement requires resources for projects, training, external help, and information processing, among other elements. A test of commitment to quality improvement is whether leaders are willing to invest significantly in the initiative.

4. *Information systems.* A fundamental aspect of quality philosophy is that data must be distributed to quality teams where they need them and when they need them. Some companies are set to deliver these data, whereas others must first develop their information systems capability. Further, most organizations need to teach their new quality teams and managers how to use the data effectively. Building an adequate information infrastructure is a critical support component because without data, the fundamental concepts of quality management are undercut.

5. *Training.* Sometimes it is assumed that new strategic initiatives can be undertaken without training. This assumption is a serious mistake in the quality management field, where tools and techniques as well as the understanding of "what works how" are expanding rapidly. An investment in training is essential for a successful quality management program and also signals to clinical and administrative staff that the effort is serious and long-lasting.

6. *Incentives.* Many organizations are incorporating into their personnel and performance-review structures incentives for participating in, and realizing, quality gains. Annual reviews of the quality contributions of clinical and administrative staff may be tied to merit and bonus pay, may provide access to new departmental resources, and may appear in the strategic plan by which all executives will be judged.

7. *Communication and feedback.* Organization leaders are realizing that communication and feedback must be provided to all participants in the quality improvement project and in the health care organization in general. This feedback sustains the quality improvement efforts, develops "buy-in" by the employees, and creates pride in the health care organization. The feedback loops are usually formalized in the quality management department by official reporting of the quality improvement project. However, all members of the organization need to understand their part in improving quality, and this understanding can be furthered through employee newsletters, survey questions, and other mechanisms.

Obstructions

Many organizations have encountered difficulties in implementing quality management. Obstructions may be found in the organization's technology, structure, psychological climate, leadership, culture, and involvement in legal issues. Each of these areas is summarized below.

1. *Technology.* Many organizations' quality managers have had to learn new quality management techniques while simultaneously building the information infrastructure needed to do the

work. In many organizations, the "technology of quality management" is relatively new and has only been lightly used and tested by the staff. In the last 10 years, strides have been made in developing a set of quality management tools and techniques that are consistent with a continuous improvement philosophy; many innovations still await widespread diffusion.

2. *Structure.* Some leaders have taken aggressive steps to put quality councils in place, to recognize quality improvement gains in public ways, and to inject quality into performance requirements. However, these efforts are by no means widespread. How to structure the quality effort, and how much visibility to give the quality initiative in the organizational structure, are two barriers that often result in inaction.

3. *Psychological climate.* The climate of the organization sometimes presents a barrier to two fundamental aspects of quality philosophy: openness to data sharing, and teamwork. Quality management requires that the staff collects and analyzes data and shares the findings in open meetings, yet the climate of some organizations is too closed for this type of exposure. In other organizations, teamwork is only an occasional proposition. Because quality improvement depends on examining relationships and interdependencies across departmental boundaries and hierarchical levels, a lack of familiarity with this "boundaryless" movement may be a barrier.

4. *Leadership.* Just as leadership can support quality management, it can also obstruct it. Unless quality management has a clear and continuous commitment from the organization's leader, the quality effort is doomed. Frequently, the leader fails to adequately communicate the importance of the quality effort and its ongoing progress. The leader must demonstrate visible support for the quality effort constantly. Clinical and administrative staffs are keenly sensitive to any real or perceived wavering of support.

5. *Culture.* In Deming's view,[4] successful quality management requires building a supportive organizational culture. Conversely, an organizational culture that has the following characteristics conflicts with the basic philosophy of quality management: decisions are made from the top down; the workforce is not empowered; communication tends to be closed (data are not openly shared); patients' interests are subservient to medical-center objectives; errors bring blame-seeking and dismissal; and teamwork is thought unnecessary. Starting quality efforts in a hostile environment is a doomed experiment. Unfortunately, many academic medical centers and large community institutions lack a history of a supportive culture for quality improvement.

6. *Legal issues.* An easy way to disable a quality program is to saddle it with legal implications. In such a climate, patients will not sign release forms, and the organization cannot legally ask for or disseminate information. Because provider contracts do not specify that data can be requested, an organization's managers must be creative and innovative in moving these legal issues aside without harming the organization, its employees, and the patients who receive care.

● Accrediting and Regulatory Oversight Organizations

Many types of accrediting and regulatory oversight organizations are active in the quality management field. Some have long histories in the health care industry, and others were established in the previous 10 to 20 years. As part of their mission, these organizations have taken on improving the quality of medical and health care services at the individual, team, unit, organization, and population levels. Instead of focusing on only one or two levels, they strive to raise the quality of care across the delivery spectrum.

Organizational Characteristics

To illustrate the contributions of accrediting and regulatory oversight organizations to quality management, organizational characteristics are described below for two leading organizations: the Joint Commission on the Accreditation of Healthcare Organizations (JCAHO) and the National Committee for Quality Assurance (NCQA), both of which accredit health care organizations (hospitals and managed care plans). The characteristics, which also are used to describe the quality roles of other oversight organizations, are purpose, targets, approach and methodology, timing, locus of control, leadership, power, and costs.[36]

1. *Purpose.* Achieving quality improvement involves two primary purposes: (1) *accountability,* with policing to protect various stakeholders, such as patients, citizens, and corporate purchasers; and (2) *organizational and practice development,* to support the intended continuous improvement of clinical and administrative systems. JCAHO reviews hospitals with both purposes in mind: policing in an accrediting sense, and development to the extent that its surveys and standards help to raise the level of patient care. NCQA also is the "accountability agent" for the managed care industry; through the use of its surveys and criteria, it intends to move plan development and management to a higher level. Although each organization incorporates both policing and development in its reviews, subjects of the reviews tend to see the policing side as dominant.

2. *Targets.* Three main potential subjects for quality review are: (1) structure, such as credentials, staffing levels, number of hospital beds, and official rules and procedures; (2) processes, such as the means and actions of providing care and support services (e.g., diagnoses, therapies, and follow-up care); and (3) outcomes or results, such as death, complications, infections, satisfaction, and functional status. In their early development, both JCAHO and NCQA focused mostly on structure, following the philosophy that if the right structures were in place, quality processes and desired outcomes would follow. However, in the 1990s, quality managers in both organizations began to look for actual data on outcomes, asking for evidence of desired improvement. In effect, they began to test the assumptions of the structure-process-outcome linkage.

3. *Approach and methodology.* Numerous combinations of approaches to quality improvement exist, from simple individual clinical-case review and screens using statistics, quality tools, and benchmarks, to continuous quality improvement using problem-solving cycles in every aspect of clinical administrative processes. Proponents of traditional quality assurance use policy and methods (such as inspection) to search for and "root out bad apples," whereas continuous quality improvement adherents see data collection and analysis, and organizational learning as the path to continuous improvement.

The primary methods used by JCAHO and NCQA are surveys and data, and outcomes analysis. In adopting these methods, the leaders of these organizations have taken the view that continuous quality improvement is based on data, facts, and information.

4. *Timing.* Several timing options are available to accrediting and regulatory oversight organizations: regular periods, such as a yearly review; occasional visits or reviews without a schedule; and continuous monitoring. Both JCAHO and NCQA use regular-visit schedules as part of their review processes. The assumption is that quality improvement work continues between visits. JCAHO is beginning a pilot program of unannounced surveys. Some accredited regulatory bodies collect data on a continuous basis from health care organizations.

5. *Locus of control.* Control of the quality improvement activity can originate with the internal unit (the department or organization) or with an external unit, such as a regulatory group or

governmental agency. Internal quality efforts are designed and driven by the clinical and administrative leaders of the service provider, and they illustrate organizational interest and investment in quality. In efforts with an external locus, the design and quality assessments are led by an external organization and "quality review specialists" who are not under the control of the provider agency.

Organizations may make quality improvement efforts that are separate from the JCAHO and NCQA requirements. Deeply committed organizations have invested in, and are committed to, quality well beyond the requirements of the accrediting groups. Because these organizations are internally driven, they see quality as a value-added contribution to their organization that extends beyond the desire to gain accreditation.

6. *Leadership.* Leadership is provided by those persons who are responsible for designing and operating quality management in the organization. In some organizations, such as hospitals or managed care plans, the CEO personally handles the liaison with the outside oversight groups (e.g., JCAHO and NCQA). Providing such liaison is an opportunity to demonstrate the depth of commitment and knowledge of the executive team. In other cases, survey teams are dismissed merely as "regulators" or "paper bureaucrats," to be satisfied at minimal cost to the clinical and business enterprise. Questions frequently asked by visitors are, "Who leads the quality effort: the medical executive, or the administrative executive?" and "Or is leadership a joint effort?"

7. *Power.* The power to encourage or force change can come from several sources, including personal power (the expertise and interest of the leadership), or structural power (the power of the position). It can also come from the legal or regulatory requirements. Many oversight organizations rely on the power of the "stamp of approval" in the marketplace. Successful reviews by JCAHO and NCQA signal to corporate purchasers—and to some extent patients (if they read the reviews)—that the organization meets or exceeds quality standards. In summary, the review teams have power to force change in quality through coercive policing. Further, they have the power to encourage developmental improvement because of the shared recognition of their expertise and leadership.

8. *Costs.* The costs are typically categorized as high, medium, or low, according to the time and personnel resources required to engage in the quality reviews. For example, high costs are involved in long-term, large sample studies of process and outcome; much lower costs would be associated with a one-time review of 30 randomly selected cases in a small group practice. The accrediting visits are costly for the organizations because of the direct costs of the review process and the indirect costs of preparation. As the demands for greater sophistication in quality management rise, so will the cost to the organization.

Key Organizations

A list of some key organizations' websites that offer quality-related services follows:

1. American Hospital Association Quality Initiative, *www.hospitalconnect.com/aha/key_issues/patient_safetyadvocacy/quality_initiative.html*
2. American Society for Healthcare Risk Management, *www.hospitalconnect.com/ashrm/aboutus/aboutus.html*
3. American Health Quality Association, *www.ahqa.org*
4. National Association for Healthcare Quality, *www.nahq.org*
5. Picker Institute, *www.pickereurope.org*

6. Quality Indicator Project, *www.qiproject.org*
7. Center for the Evaluative Clinical Sciences at Dartmouth, *www.dartmouth.edu/~cecs*

Summary

The success and failure of total quality improvement and continuous quality management rest in the culture of the organization and in the participation of the key stakeholders of the delivery system. Traditionally, medical care has been organized in a rigid, top-down system, with the physician as the decisionmaker. However, if outcomes are to improve, all caregivers must participate in decisionmaking. Other forces, such as purchasers, regulators, consumers and accrediting bodies, are also insisting on the use of outcomes to identify quality.

Health care is moving to a system that is based on measuring defined outcomes for individuals and populations. Evidence-based medicine is being identified as the process that can best decrease the variation in the practice of medicine on an individual and organizational basis. Quality is becoming the responsibility of the health care community at large, not just of the quality assurance department. In all health care organizations, quality is being appropriately driven from the top down, with feedback loops and integrated teamwork. *Measurement* and *metrics* have become the new bywords.

Persuading individual practitioners to change practice patterns has been difficult despite incentives, information, collegiality, reprimand, and other techniques. Yet all stakeholders of health care—providers, purchasers, patients, and suppliers—must be included if quality care is to be the mainstay of the health care delivery system. Finally, quality managers must confront the issue of the interface between cost and quality. Today, the cost of health care is paramount to most purchasers, and quality managers need to prove that quality, rather than cost, is the appropriate choice.

Quality is the most important issue in health care today. In *Crossing the Quality Chasm: A New Health System for the 21st Century*, the Institute of Medicine has identified 13 major recommendations that should be addressed in order to enable the United States to develop the quality health care system it needs and deserves.[36]

References

1. Codman E. The product of a hospital. *Surgical and Gynecology and Obstetrics.* 1914.
2. Donabedian A. *The Methods and Findings of Quality Assessment and Monitoring, Volumes I, II, III.* Ann Arbor, MI: Health Administration Press; 1985.
3. Juran JM. *Juran on Leadership for Quality.* New York, NY: Free Press; 1989.
4. Deming WE. *Out of the Crisis.* Cambridge, MA: Center for Advanced Engineering Study; 1982.
5. Crosby PB. *Quality Is Free: The Art of Making Quality Certain.* New York, NY: McGraw-Hill; 1979.
6. Chassin MR, Galvin RW. The urgent need to improve health care quality. *Institute of Medicine National Roundtable on Health Care Quality* [review: 41 refs]. *JAMA.* 1998;280(11):1000–1005.
7. Committee on Quality of Health Care in America, Institute of Medicine. Kohn LT, Corrigan JM, Donaldson MS (eds). *To Err Is Human: Building a Safer Health System.* Washington, DC: National Academy Press; 2000. Available at: *http://books.nap.edu/books/0309068371/html/index.html.*
8. Committee on Quality of Health Care in America, Institute of Medicine. *Crossing the Quality Chasm: A New Health System for the 21st Century.* Washington, DC: National Academy Press; 2001. Available at: *http://books.nap.edu/books/0309072808/html/index.html.*

9. Silimperi DR, Franco LM, Veldhuyzen van Zanten T, MacAulay C. A framework for institutionalizing quality assurance. *Int J Qual Health Care.* 2002;14 (suppl 1:67–73):(13).

10. Mohr JJ, Mahoney CC, Nelso ED, Batalden PB, Plume SK. Improving health care, Part 3: Clinical benchmarking for best patient care. *Joint Com J Qual Improv.* 1996;22(9):599-616.

11. Kiefe CI, Weissman NW, Allison JJ, Farmer R, Weaver M, Williams OD. Identifying achievable benchmarks of care: Concepts and methodology. *Int J Qual Health Care.* 1998;10(5):443–447.

12. Dean JW, Evans, JR. *Total Quality: Management, Organization, and Strategy.* St. Paul, MN: West Group; 1994.

13. Gerard JC, Arnold FL. Performance improvement with a hybrid FOCUS-PDCA methodology. *Jt Comm J Qual Improv.* 1996;22(10):41,660–672.

14. Nelson EC, Johr JJ, Batalden PB, Plume SK. Improving health care, part 1: The clinical value compass. *Jt Comm J Qual Improv.* 1996;22(4):42,243–258.

15. Bates DW, Pappius E, Kuperman GJ, et al. Partners Information Systems, Boston, MA 02115, USA. *Int J Med Inf.* 1999;53(2–3):115–124.

16. Weingart SN, Iezzoni LI, Davis RB, et al. Use of administrative data to find substandard care: Validation of the complications screening program. *Med Care.* 2000;38(8):53,796–806.

17. Dranove D, Reynolds KS, Gillies RR, Shortell SS, Rademaker AW, Huang CF. The cost of efforts to improve quality. *Med Care.* 1999;37(10);1084–1087.

18. Iezzoni LI. The risks of risk adjustment. *JAMA.* 1997;278(19):1600–1607.

19. Khuri SF, Daley J, Henderson W, et al. Relation of surgical volume to outcome in eight common operations: Results from the VA National Surgical Quality Improvement Program. *Ann Surg.* 1999;230(3): 414–429;discussion,429–432.

20. Maryland Medicaid Program Risk Adjustment Methodology.

21. *The Economist,* June 11, 1998, p. 72.

22. Committee on the National Quality Report on Health Care Delivery, Institute of Medicine. Corrigan JM, Hurtado MP, Swift EK (eds.). *Envisioning the National Health Care Quality Report.* Washington, DC: National Academy Press; 2001.

23. Dull VT, Lansky D, Davis N. Evaluating a patient satisfaction survey for maximum benefit. *Joint Com J Qual Improv.* 1994;20(8):444–453.

24. Bigby M. Evidence-based medicine in a nutshell. A guide to finding and using the best evidence in caring for patients. *Arch Dermotol.* 1998;134(12):120,1609–1618.

25. Powell C. The Delphi technique: Myths and realities. *J Adv Nurs.* 2003;41(4):376–382.

26. Grilli R, Magrini N, Penna A, Mura G, Liberati A. Practice guidelines developed by specialty societies: The need for a critical appraisal. *Lancet.* 2000;355(9198):103–106.

27. *www.ncqa.org*

28. *www.healthypeople.gov*

29. *www.dmaa.org*

30. Chassin MR. Achieving and sustaining improved quality: Lessons from New York State and cardiac surgery. *Health Aff (Millwood).* 2002;21(4):40–51,119.

31. Fox R. Quality improvement: Leaders needed. *Circulation.* 2002;106(23):e9064–9065.

32. Sackett DL, Rosenberg WM. The need for evidence-based medicine. *J R Soc Med.* 1995;88(11):120,620–624.

33. Miles-Doan R, Kelly S. Inequities in health care and survival after injury among pedestrians: Explaining the urban/rural differential. *J Rural Health.* 1995;11(3):121,177–184.

34. Wennberg D, Dickens J Jr, Soule D et al. The relationship between the supply of cardiac catheterization laboratories, cardiologists and the use of invasive cardiac procedures in northern New England. *J Health Serv Res Policy.* 1997;2(2):75–80,121.

35. Ziegenfuss JT. Policies for quality of care in medical and healthcare organizations in Quebec: The diversity of options and actors. *Canadian J. Quality Health Care.* 1997;14(1):15–20.

36. Focus newsletter of the American College of Medical Quality. May–June 2003;13(3).

● Web Sites for Health Care Quality

The following list, compiled by the author, includes web sites for established organizations that are involved in health care quality. It is not exhaustive but represents many well-respected and well-known researchers and authorities on health care quality:

Agency for Healthcare Research and Quality—*www.ahrq.gov*

Joint Commission on Accreditation of Healthcare Organizations—*www.jcaho.org*

National Committee for Quality Assurance—*www.ncqa.org*

National Quality Forum—*www.qualityforum.org*

Quality and Safety in Healthcare—*www.qhc.bmjjournals.com*

Medicare (Centers for Medicare and Medicaid Services)—*www.medicare.gov*

National Association for Healthcare Quality—*www.nahq.org*

The American Health Quality Association—*www.ahqa.org*

Institute for Healthcare Improvement—*www.ihi.org*

Foundation for Health Care Quality—*www.qualityhealth.org*

FACCT (Foundation for Accountability)- *www.facct.org*

Health Resources and Services Administration—*www.ask.hrsa.gov/quality.cfm*

Institute of Medicine Quality Initiative—*www.iom.edu/IOM/IOMHome.nsf/pages/quality+Initiative*

The American College of Medical Quality—*www.acmq.org*

URAC—*www.urac.org*

Quality Interagency Coordination Task Force (QuIC)—*www.quic.gov*

Rand Health—*www.rand.org/health*

Kaiser Family Foundation—*www.kaisernetwork.org*

Addendum

Institute of Medicine Reports
Composite Summary

Prepared by the ACMQ Medical Informatics Forum

This summary aims to provide an overview of the reports published by the Institute of Medicine (IOM) over the past three years.
The relevant IOM reports are:
- To Err is Human: Building a Safer Health System[1]
- Crossing the Quality Chasm: A New Health System for the 21st Century[2]
- Envisioning a National Healthcare Quality Report[3]
- Leadership by Example: Coordinating Government Roles in Improving Health Care Quality[4]
- Priority Area for National Action: Transforming Health Care Quality[5]

TO ERR IS HUMAN
This report deals with system errors and adverse events

The report's recommendations include:
- Establish a mandatory system for reporting errors and adverse events;
- Designate the National Forum for Health Care Quality Measurement and Reporting (National Quality Forum) to set reporting standards;
- Require health care organizations to report;
- Require states to establish reporting systems and set performance standards and expectations for safety.

These recommendations are directed at health care organizations, health care professionals and professional licensure boards, regulators, accreditors and purchasers, professional societies and the FDA.
Additional recommendations include:
- Encourage regulatory and accreditation organizations to require patient safety programs;
- Encourage private and public purchasers to provide incentives to health care organizations;
- Require licensing bodies to implement re-examination and re-licensure of professionals;
- Develop curriculum for patient safety;
- Disseminate information on patient safety and incorporate the data into clinical practice guidelines;
- Establish community-based collaborative initiatives;
- Redesign drug packaging and labeling;
- Modify drug naming;
- Establish post-marketing surveillance;
- Provide visible attention;
- Implement non-punitive systems;
- Establish team-training programs;
- Incorporate well-understood safety principles;
- Implement proven medication safety practices.

CROSSING THE QUALITY CHASM
This report identifies gaps in the delivery of patient care services

An agenda to "cross the chasm" includes the need for leadership to facilitate change, the need to commit to a statement of purpose and the adoption of a new set of principles. A strong case is made to identify a set of priority conditions that should be the focus of attention. The need to design and implement organizational support for changes is tied to the efforts that are needed to foster and reward improvement. The recommendations recognize the requirement to prepare the workforce for a world of expanding knowledge and rapid change. The report recommends the creation of an information infrastructure to support evidenced-based decision-making by patients and members of the healthcare delivery team.
Six "aims for improvement" are articulated and these are:
- A system that is safe;
- A system that is designed to avoid injury;
- Services that are effective, i.e. based on scientific knowledge and patient centered;
- Services that are timely;
- Services that are delivered efficiently;
- Services that are delivered in an equitable manner.

New principles and rules for design of care are described, with the centerpiece being a commitment to care that is evidence-based, patient centered, and systems-based.
Some principles and framework for effecting change include an understanding of complex adaptive systems integrated with the characteristics of a learning organization. The concept that access to information and the transfer of knowledge can be defined as "care" drive many of the recommendations. It is recognized that rules will occasionally conflict and should not be taken to the extreme.

The new principles and rules for design of care include the establishment of a continuous healing relationship, with a 24 hours a day/7 days week/365 days a year commitment. These design features require customization based on patient needs and values, with the patient as the source of control. Such relationships will be facilitated by sharing knowledge, by the free flow of information, and by the use of evidence-based decision-making.

New principles and rules for design of care have the following features:

- Safety as a system property;
- Transparency;
- Anticipation of needs;
- Decrease of waste;
- Cooperation among practitioners.

There is a need to focus on the 80/20 rule. The report notes that 20 percent of patients account for 80 percent of work in delivering care and account for a similar percentage of the costs of care. Similarly, 20 percent of diagnoses account for 80 percent of the health problems of the population. A concentration on usual care while planning for contingencies will serve the population well.

Steps toward systems improvement:

- Focus on the fifteen priority conditions: cancer, diabetes, emphysema, high cholesterol, HIV/AIDS, hypertension, ischemic heart disease, stroke, arthritis, asthma, gall bladder disease, stomach ulcers, back problems, Alzheimer's, other dementias, depression and anxiety;
- Organize processes around these conditions, basing processes on evidence-based best practices;
- Create the necessary information infrastructure to support provision of care;
- Practice ongoing measurement of care processes;
- Align the incentives of the various stakeholders.

Organizational challenges included the need to redesign care processes and the steps that must be taken to facilitate the effective use of information technologies. A critical success factor will be the recognition of the growing knowledge gap and ways to manage it, including the application of new tools and the provision of training of healthcare professionals in the new skills required. Changes in licensure and continuous professional development, including fostering life-long learning, are integral components of the changes needed.

Changes to the payment policy and workforce mix must occur. Coordination across patient conditions, services and settings is an essential component of the new system, as are efforts to advance the effectiveness of teams delivering care.

ENVISIONING A NATIONAL HEALTH CARE QUALITY REPORT

This report addresses the collection, measurement and analysis of quality data

The report:

- Provides a framework for the content of a data set needed to support the measurement of quality;
- Outlines a process for selecting the measurements;
- Provides an analysis of data sources;
- Defines report formats.

Two dimensions of quality are highlighted, one being the "medical" model and the second being from the patient's perspective.

The Medical Model

The dimensions of the medical model include safety, effectiveness, "patient centeredness," and timelines, as well as equity and effectiveness.

Patient centeredness encompasses the relationship between the patient and clinicians, implies a partnership between patient and healthcare professionals, and requires ensuring that decisions respect the patient's needs and preferences. Further attributes include taking into account the patient's experience with care, and embedding into the relationship caring, a commitment to open communication and efforts to understand the patient's needs. An effective partnership includes shared decision-making, with the incorporation of opportunities for self-monitoring, goal setting and the accrual of skills and knowledge to provide for self-management.

The Patient's Perspective

This section, for the purposes of describing a measurement set, identifies patients into four areas:

- Staying healthy;
- Getting better;
- Living with illness/disability; and
- Coping with end of life.

Selection of Measures

- The criteria for selecting the measures should include overall importance, impact on health, and meaningfulness.
- The measures should be influenced by the systems or the entities being measured.
- The selected measures should be scientifically sound, valid, reliable and based on evidence.
- Collection of data must have feasibility, which means availability of data across sources and systems, at reasonable costs, without a significant data collection burden.
- The measures should have the capacity to support subgroup analysis.
- Prototypes for these measures should exist.
- Summary measures are not encouraged, but when used should be within the same dimension.
- An appropriate balance between outcome-validated process measures and conditions/procedure specific

outcome measures, strongly linked by evidence, is recommended.

- Structural measures should be avoided

Report Design

The report comments extensively on the design needs of a national report:

- The need to tailor the reports to different users;
- The need to limit the number of key findings and measures that should be included in the report because of the evidence of the limited ability of end users to process information.
- The use of benchmarks;
- Inclusion of findings with strong statistical evidence and those that are actionable;
- Regular updates;
- The use of sidebars to highlight stories and engage the reader emotionally.
- Pre-testing and assessing how the report can be used by the public.

LEADERSHIP BY EXAMPLE

This report addresses the duplication and disparate approaches to performance measures by government agencies

Obstacles to a successful system:

- Lack of consistency in performance measures because of multiple existing efforts;
- Increased data collections burden because of multiple existing efforts;
- Lack of a conceptual framework to guide performance measure selection;
- Lack of access to computerized clinical data;
- Lack of a commitment to transparency;
- Lack of availability of comparative quality data in the public domain;
- Absence of a systematic approach for assessing the impact of QI projects conducted in various settings.

"Big picture" recommendations include:

- Collaboration between the six federal programs – Medicare, Medicaid, DOD, VA, Tricare and the Indian Health Service – in their efforts to develop standardized sets of performance measures;
- Collaboration in the federal programs' collection of clinical data to support the performance measures;
- Provision of incentives, including financial incentives, to encourage the collection of the necessary data;
- A commitment to building the IT infrastructure needed to support measurement and decision-making;
- The creation of a performance measure data repository;
- A commitment for federal entities such as the VA and DOD to serve as laboratories;
- The creation of conduits through which to disseminate information;

- Collaboration with the private sector;
- Support for the conduct of research.

Additional recommendations (expanded) include:

- Establishment of quality expectations;
- Consumer participation: raise awareness of quality gap, facilitate input into measurement design, secure assessments of care, facilitate selection, including selection of treatment options;
- Establishment of clinical data reporting requirements;
- Purchasing strategies;
- Identification of best practices;
- Release of public domain comparative quality data;
- Establishment of public programs to act as delivery system models and dissemination of the findings;
- Creation of public domain IT products;
- Requirement that AHRQ and others pursue applied research, develop new knowledge and tools to support quality enhancement;
- Requirement that QuIC promulgate standardized performance measures for five conditions by 2003 and ten conditions by 2004;
- Coordination with the six federal programs for roll-out by 2008;
- Private sector providers to be informed of the need to submit audited patient level data (Medicare, Medicaid, SCHIP and portions of Tricare);
- Government providers (VA, DOD and portions of Tricare) to be required to prepare immediately;
- IT infrastructure to be developed for quality enhancement, bioterrorism surveillance, public health and research;
- Congressional consideration to rapid development IT infrastructure by tax incentives, (loans and grants);
- Adoption of regulatory and market driven approaches to encourage investment (rapid payment, COP);
- Reliance on web-based technology;
- Requirement that software and intellectual property be in the public domain.

PRIORITY AREAS FOR NATIONAL ACTION

This report identifies priorities from the earlier reports and suggests a framework for action

Four stages of life and health are described in the four circles, connected by the need for co-ordination across time and healthcare delivery settings.

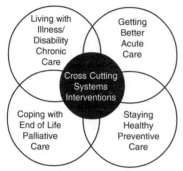

The criteria used for the conditions and topics selected for highest priority focus included:

- **Impact**
  Considerations were degree of disability, mortality and economic consequences.
- **Improvability**
  Considerations focused on supporting literature (evidence) concerning the likelihood for improvement, and on the likelihood of achieving the previously stated six national aims: safety, effectiveness, patient-centeredness, timeliness, efficiency and equity.
- **Inclusiveness**
  Considerations were activities across populations and settings.

The twenty priority areas recommended are (in no particular order):

- Asthma
- Cancer screening (colorectal and cervical)
- Diabetes
- Hypertension
- Ischemic heart disease
- Major depression
- Stroke
- Medication management (errors and overuse antibiotics)
- Nosocomial infections
- Pregnancy and childbirth
- Mental illness
- End of life organ failure
- Immunizations
- Frailty associated with old age
- Pain control
- Care coordination
- Tobacco dependence
- Self-management / health literacy
- Children with special needs
- Obesity

References:

1. Committee on Quality of Health Care in America, Institute of Medicine. Kohn LT, Corrigan JM, Donaldson MS (eds.). (2000). To err is human: building a safer health system. Washington, DC: National Academy Press.
   This report can be viewed online at http://books.nap.edu/ books/0309068371/html/index.html

2. Committee on Quality of Health Care in America, Institute of Medicine. (2001). Crossing the quality chasm: a new health system for the 21st century. Washington, DC: National Academy Press.
   This report can be viewed online at http://books.nap.edu/ books/0309072808/html/index.html

3. Committee on the National Quality Report on Health Care Delivery, Institute of Medicine. Corrigan JM, Hurtado MP, Swift EK, (eds.). (2001). Envisioning the national health care quality report. Washington, DC: National Academy Press.
   This report can be viewed online at http://search.nap.edu/ books/030907343X/html

4. Committee on Enhancing Federal Quality Healthcare Programs. Corrigan JM, Eden J, Smith BM (eds.). (2002). Leadership by example: coordinating government roles in improving health care quality. Washington, DC: National Academy Press.
   This report can be viewed online at http://www.nap.edu/ books/0309086183/html

5. Committee on Identifying Areas for Quality Improvement, Institute of Medicine, Board on Health Care Services. Adams K, Corrigan JM (eds.). (2003). Priority areas for national action: transforming health care quality. Washington, DC: National Academy Press.
   This report can be viewed online at http://books.nap.edu/ books/0309085438/html/index.html

Chapter 2

UTILIZATION MANAGEMENT

Eric Z. Silfen, MD, MSHA

Ralph H Rosenblum, Jr., DDS, MHA

Introduction

Utilization management is an essential component in a comprehensive program of medical services that are planned, implemented, evaluated, and monitored to meet health care needs in a high-quality and cost-effective manner. As defined by the Utilization Review Accreditation Commission (URAC; *www.urac.org*), utilization review is "a process, performed by or on behalf of a third-party payer that evaluates the medical necessity, appropriateness, and efficiency of the use of health care services, procedures, and facilities."[1] In addition, utilization management compares the characteristics of specific clinical care to predetermined or established protocols and benchmarks that are derived from external standards or from internal comparison among aggregate case groups.[2] These evaluations can be performed as part of peer review, administrative review, or public or private agency review.[3] Finally, in addition to clarifying process management, compliance with regulatory requirements, and appropriate metric selection, utilization management depends on the accuracy and reliability of patient care information.[4]

Six concepts guide the utilization management discussion:

1. Background purpose of utilization management
2. Developmental milestones in utilization management
3. Methods and procedures of utilization management
4. Outcomes and benefits of utilization management
5. Organizational structures that enable—and barriers that interfere with—utilization management
6. Accreditation and regulatory organizations involved in utilization management

Development of Utilization Management

Background and Purpose

The necessity for utilization management to be a component of medical decisionmaking was summarized in a commentary published in 2001 in the *Journal of the American Medical Association*. The article stated, in part:

> The United States faces an accelerating demand for medical services due to new quality-enhancing but cost increasing drugs and devices, an ever-broadening social definition of health, and an ever more informed and assertive consumer. Despite unprecedented prosperity, the nation lacks the economic resources to finance all services that would provide some benefit to some patient. The setting of social priorities and balancing of competing claims is imperative. The fundamental question concerns where and by whom these difficult decisions will be made. Five candidates present themselves: government, employers, insurers, physicians, and consumers. Each has serious limitations as arbiter of who should get what, yet of necessity one must be assigned the role.

Utilization management, or utilization review, began in the 1970s as a mechanism to evaluate medical costs after services had been provided. In the 1980s, most utilization management was still retrospective. However, the impetus shifted from a purely paper, claim-based evaluation to include telephone inquiry information. The use of the telephone was the harbinger of prospective decisionmaking, such as pre-certification, as well as the concurrent review of medical practice. Currently, utilization management combines retrospective, concurrent, and prospective reviews.[5]

The 1970s experienced the beginning of state regulation of utilization management to address practitioner concerns about the validity and fairness of utilization management programs. Currently, 35 states require health care organizations that receive public funds to meet utilization management standards. These standards must be flexible enough to permit appropriate, case-by-case variations. In addition, some states incorporated utilization management into the regulations of the workers' compensation administration, as well as in-hospital, third party, and individual practitioner evaluations.[6]

In the early 1990s, concern about utilization management programs was sufficient enough to establish the Utilization Review Accreditation Commission (URAC). The Commission is a nonprofit organization that sets standards for various aspects of health care delivery, such as case management, health plan operation, workers' compensation claims management, health insurance claims management, health call-center operation, and health information web sites.[7]

As activity in utilization management became prospective and concurrent, rather than retrospective, the term "utilization management" became more widely used than "utilization review." During this transition, complementary disease management programs, case management programs, and care management programs were incorporated into utilization management. Standards, principally developed by URAC, were instituted to require specific timelines for medical and administrative determinations, as well as for the appeal and grievance processes. At the end of the 1990s, groups independent of the third-party payer organizations instituted requirements for external review to provide an additional level of oversight.[8]

Developmental Milestones

1. *Cost pressure.* During the 1980s and 1990s, health care organizations faced driving forces from outside their organizational boundaries. The increasing cost of health care made hospital leaders sensitive to financing services; insurance companies and insurance plans; corporate buyers of health care

services; and politicians from local, state and federal levels. This greatly-enhanced sensitivity to the cost resulted in utilization management being recognized as a tool for restraining and managing costs.[9]

2. *Interest in quality improvement.* During the late 1980s and 1990s, interest in quality improvement methodologies and approaches increased. There was a strong belief that health care organizations could assess the quality of medical care by examining the resources used in providing that care. Additionally, variation in resource utilization was identified as both a quality-of-service issue and a conservation imperative. Not only could attention be paid to utilization for the purpose of controlling costs, but utilization indicators could raise quality questions and help with judgments about the quality of care.[10]

3. *Methodological development.* Early efforts to engage in utilization management were basic and fundamental. During the last several decades, structurally sophisticated and data-intensive methodologies and approaches have been developed, resulting in an increase in breadth and scope of utilization management programs.[11]

4. *Information systems support.* Following the methodological developments, the foundation for utilization management was broadened by the recognition of the need for information system support, substantial investments in information system development, and widely increased organizational capabilities. The use of computer-based information technologies and the availability of data on clinical outcomes, patient records, practitioner and facility services, and costs have substantially changed utilization management activities. Along with improved information systems and technology, e-mail communication and computer submission of claims data became common, shortening the time required for utilization management activities.

5. *Incremental acceptance.* Although clinicians' acceptance of utilization management may be reluctant, many recognize that utilization management is an essential component of patient care. In addition, more clinicians have been exposed to strategic and organizational decisionmaking, giving them the opportunity to recognize the need to control and conserve resources more carefully. Utilization management departments also have made substantial contributions to organizational missions and goals, and the concurrent knowledge gains have impressed clinicians.[12]

6. *Demonstrated impact.* Utilization management professionals must firmly believe that the programs will make a positive contribution. Fortunately, the positive contributions of the utilization management programs in supporting patient-centered health care have been numerous, such as (1) consensus guideline approach to hospital services; (2) reduction in hospital admission and readmission rates; and (3) pharmaceutical savings. As a matter of strategic policy, organizations promote awareness of these contributions, whereas others expect the impact of utilization management to gradually gain traction within the organization.[13]

To maximize clinical outcomes and patient satisfaction (and to paraphrase medication safety jargon,) utilization management depends on the delivery of care according to the five patient rights: (1) the right care (2) to the right patient (3) in the right amount (4) at the right time, and (5) in the right environment.[69]

In conjunction with this process emphasis, six factors emerge as critical for the development and growth of utilization management programs:

1. The increase in published benchmark data, such as data from the Health Plan Employer Data and Information Set (HEDIS), practitioner profiles, and physician "report cards," has raised the standards of care simply by making utilization comparisons easily accessible to the consumer.

2. Changes in medical technology are occurring faster than hardware and applications can be evaluated. Although this situation provides job security for quality and utilization managers, it forces utilization management programs to be ongoing processes that must mature to keep pace with current progress.[15]

3. The electronic patient record offers advantages for utilization managers. Computerized access to patient-level data allows precise analyses of patient care. Simultaneously, the privacy and confidentiality of protected health information (PHI), through the Health Insurance Portability and Accountability Act (HIPAA), new privacy laws, and emerging legal precedents delineates the required strict controls over who has access to patient-level data, at what time, and for what purpose. Therefore, utilization management programs should evolve to incorporate these patient-privacy protections and medical-record confidentiality requirements.

4. As quality oversight and monitoring mechanisms become integrated into utilization management programs, improved processes have made medical necessity determinations more efficient.[14] As managed care companies move toward a coordination-of-care model, utilization management should be less rigid in applying pre-certification and concurrent review requirements. Because this model moves beyond actuarially based, predictive, decisionmaking criteria and focuses on accountability for outcomes of care, the traditional utilization management models formulated on retrospective data have limited capability to address emerging disease management and patient management goals.[27] In addition, the flexibility inherent in emerging utilization management models will incorporate evidence-based medicine guidelines, as well as clinical and patient satisfaction outcomes that are as important as cost and resource utilization control.[29]

5. Utilization management systems will have greater inter-observer reliability regarding patient care decisions.[32] As managerial systems will be more efficient, determinations regarding admissions or procedures will be more expeditious. In addition, the increase in real-time decisionmaking can support customized utilization management programs that reflect payer needs. At the same time, patients and consumers can become more involved in managing their care as they learn more about their health conditions and treatment options.[28] Both disease management programs and information retrievable from Web-enabled applications will fuel these changes.[67] Because managerial systems have improved grievance and appeals processes, as well as quality monitoring mechanisms, the application of information technology to regulatory demands has lead to a more open and rapid set of operational procedures.

6. Ensuring the integrity of the utilization management process is difficult when a decision to deny care is based on conflicting medical and benefit-coverage factors. This problem also arises when a procedure is denied or not certified as a request for either a second opinion or for an evaluation of an alternative treatment. The denial of payment may be consistent with health plan policies and procedures, but it may not be appropriate if the delay jeopardizes patient care. The time involved with evaluating additional opinions or alternative procedures may effectively deny service when the delay renders the original request moot.

Purpose and Perspective of Utilization Management

Utilization management is a formal examination of resource use in the various stages of patient care—primary care, emergency care, acute care, long-term care, hospice care—by means of retrospective, concurrent, or prospective methods.[30,33,36] The objective is to understand the reasons for, as well as to reduce variation in, utilization by "pulling and pushing" practitioners toward the best practices.

The goals for utilization management programs are:[26]

1. To promote, develop, and support the efficient use of patient care resources
2. To develop and implement resource utilization indicators and metrics
3. To review patient care processes
4. To design and develop information support for staff and committees
5. To create a culture of transparency by opening processes and procedures to external review and continuous development

Unfortunately, physicians and other practitioners *do not* tend to adopt uniform resource utilization for common, similar procedures. Key reasons include:

1. 80% to 90% of common medical practices have only limited scientific support in the literature[34]
2. Much of the applicable scientific research is not immediately available to medical practitioners
3. Even limited scientific information may overwhelm the processing capacity of the practitioner
4. Practitioners are inherently fallible information processors
5. Differences in observation ("measurement" error) among practitioners can lead to differences in assessment and treatment

The complexity of utilization management originates from the intertwining of clinical information, health care processes, practitioner behavior, and education, as well as general questions regarding the science of medicine.[35] In addition, the practice of offering practitioners incentives to limit resource use is controversial, has generated negative comments from patients and the news media, and has contributed to the difficulty in managing these programs.

The processes of utilization management differ little in application in hospitals, managed care plans, and private practitioner practices.[31] Common among these settings is the focus on quality of patient care and fiscal responsibility.[37] Quality of care is the core purpose for all practitioners and is affected by the health care system. Fiscal responsibility is essential for all practitioners, regardless of tax-paying status.[39] Specifically, utilization management can contribute by:

1. Promoting efficient and appropriate use of health care resources
2. Decreasing administrative and overhead costs
3. Maintaining quality care
4. Identifying length-of-stay benchmarks
5. Identifying poorly performing practitioners
6. Decreasing the micro-management of practitioner behavior
7. Determining other opportunities for savings or improvement
8. Rewarding practitioners who achieve and maintain high quality and fiscal efficiency

Differences among hospital, managed care, and private-practice practitioners reflect specific-stakeholder utilization management administrative and financial perspectives.[38] Under the Prospective Payment System, hospitals strive to provide services at a cost below the reimbursement rate set by the government.[40] Hospitals often focus on practitioner performance relative to average cost per discharge. Medical care should be necessary and sufficient to prevent waste, adverse events, or readmissions, which tend to generate costs, not revenue. Thus, hospitals are concerned with interdepartmental efficiencies and coordination, report turnaround times, ensuring that the care setting and personnel are adequate for each patient, and providing the best outcomes in the shortest time. In contrast, managed care cost structures promote the development of wellness and prevention programs, as well as practitioner practice profiles to decrease unnecessary hospitalization. Finally, because the financial structure of private-practice practitioners focuses on income maximization, justification of the appropriateness of clinical services is essential.

Finally, ethical issues in utilization management must be considered. Ideally, utilization management data should provide feedback that promotes better practice. *Data should not be used punitively.* Published benchmarks should indicate the acceptable range of performance and explain the factors that affect these findings. The performance of individual practitioners should always be thoroughly discussed before implementing any action plans. Practitioners need to understand that the purpose of utilization management programs is to assist in improving their clinical services within the confines of fiscal responsibility and not to threaten their professional standing or employment.[24]

The Process of Utilization Management

Despite increasing attention to program standardization and accreditation, there is no "best way" to perform utilization management. Each organization's utilization management effort is unique and accounts for the individual characteristics of patient populations, organizational culture, and community values.

Program Design and Work Plan

A utilization management effort usually proceeds with a *program design* and *work plan* that varies in emphasis from service to cost orientation. Some utilization management programs are developed using extensive planning processes. Others are initiated with minimal formal planning and originate from learning by doing. The extent to which a utilization management program is formalized is a function of the organizational culture and management style. However, regardless of developmental origin, most programs incorporate strategic statements (goals) and operational details (data collection methods). Generically, a utilization management program design incorporates the following elements:[41,46,48]

1. The intention to develop a utilization management program with an agreement on a process for bringing the program into existence
2. A vision and design for the utilization management effort
3. The database definition for present metrics of resource use, including: (1) industry standards, (2) competitor metrics, and (3) internal, departmental metrics
4. A comparison of the current and desired utilization management efforts, including specific identification of the gaps between present and future resource-use metrics (opportunities for improvement)
5. The strategies and action plans designed to enhance efficient resource use throughout the health plan, hospital organization, or practice
6. The action plan implementation process

7. An evaluation process for checking the progress and organizational impact of the utilization management effort

To garner support from clinical and administrative leadership, work plans for utilization management departments should address the following 10 questions:

1. What is the philosophy and general approach of the utilization management department regarding inspection, review, and continuous development? Are policies established? Is there a written plan?

2. What is the relationship of the utilization management program to senior leadership?

3. Who is the utilization management leader? What is his or her organizational position, professional qualifications, and experiential training?

4. What is the organizational structure of the utilization management program? Is an advisory committee or counsel delegated? Are utilization review teams required?

5. What are the utilization review operational constituents, including procedures, techniques and methods, quantitative versus qualitative orientation, pilot programs, computer support, staff participants, and sample accomplishments?

6. Who will staff the utilization management program?

7. What are the start-up processes, activities, and time lines?

8. Will external assistance be required to initiate the program?

9. What is the cost structure of the utilization management program, including the internal rate of return, return on investment, cost of inappropriate use, and contribution margin of the program?

10. How do utilization management leaders plan to evaluate the utilization management program? Is periodic review and assessment planned?

The Utilization Management Committee

Utilization management programs function with an advisory committee comprised of critical stakeholders and professionals with expertise in the utilization review process. Although this committee often has different charters and structures, four functions are essential:

1. Design and development or planning:
   a. Program structural design
   b. Identification of opportunities for improvement
   c. Identification of performance indicators and metrics
   d. Identification of organizational resources
   e. Alignment with the organizational strategic plan

2. Monitoring the review activity:
   a. Review progress of initiatives
   b. Develop senior leadership reports
   c. Track accreditation preparation

3. Communication with appropriate internal and external stakeholders:
   a. Resource utilization progress
   b. Program impact to work force and senior leadership
   c. Hold internal "public" meetings to present results

    d. Recognize and reward group and individual efforts

    e. Organize public celebration of progress and accomplishment

4. Program evaluation:

    a. Develop utilization management program evaluation measures

    b. Ensure accountability for program goals and objectives

    c. Present oral and written impact reports

Levels of Inquiry

Utilization management programs can be instituted at various levels of inquiry.[42] Comprehensive programs include the:

Individual

Team

Unit

Organization

Community

Example: Clinical and administrative leadership is concerned about resource utilization for coronary artery bypass graft surgery. At the *individual* level, a pilot project evaluates the performance of individual surgeons. Good physician and procedural resource utilization metrics compare individual surgeons against peer benchmarks or health plan competitors willing to share information. If leadership desires, the level of inquiry could be expanded to evaluate several aspects of cardiac surgical services provided by the *team* responsible for the coronary artery bypass graft procedure. Examples of this expanded inquiry include antibiotic use during the procedure, surgical or cardiopulmonary pump time, and staffing requirements.[43]

After the cardiac service review is completed, the utilization management staff examines the contribution of resource utilization by cardiac services relative to the *organization* as a whole. This comparison includes an assessment of revenues generated relative to resources consumed. In addition, the review evaluates the depth and breadth of cardiac services in the organization relative to competing hospitals or to industry benchmarks. At this level, utilization management becomes tactical in nature, closely allied to the strategic planning process.

Finally, utilization management staff reviews the organization's delivery of cardiac services relative to the needs of the *community*. Staff members examine how their organization meets the need for cardiac services in their community relative to other communities in the region, state, or nation. At this level of inquiry, review is intended to determine whether use of services by the population of potential patients in the community is above, below, or at the level of comparison communities. From this type of review, utilization management leaders can determine whether citizens in a community have access to the resources needed for a full range of medical and health care services.[44]

Methods

The set of utilization management methods includes:

1. Design of benefits: options structure (insurance design)
2. Demand management
3. Gatekeeping
4. Practice profiling
5. Case management

6. Preauthorization

7. Second opinion

8. Discharge planning

9. Health prevention and promotion

10. Utilization review studies

Design of Benefits: Options Structure (Insurance Design)[51,52]

Utilization management should primarily address inappropriate use of services fostered by the access-to-care model. Different practitioners and service delivery sites may promote underuse, overuse, or misuse of services, depending on the care model. The options structure or insurance design reflects an effort to control this variation in use. The purpose of options structuring as a utilization management tool is to control resource use through the design of the insurance structure. For example, by structuring options, utilization managers could limit health plan liability for patients selecting physicians who do not participate in the patients' health plans. Although choice is still available to patients, they cannot visit any practitioner they desire.

The classifications for option structures are open- and closed-panel designs. A closed-panel design restricts patients from seeing physicians not affiliated with the health plan "panel." An open-panel design allows patients to see practitioners outside the health plan panel of affiliated practitioners, although some restrictions are applicable.

Demand Management[50]

As practitioners become involved with at-risk contracts, their awareness of the use and expectations of services and the risk of financial loss is tantamount. Demand management is a prospective utilization tool that allows clinical and administrative leaders to understand the use and financial characteristics of their contracted practitioner group. For example, health plan senior leadership needs to know the factors that influence use of services—patient economic level, age, occupation, gender, race, education, health status, public coverage, and location. If these factors act as barriers to services, access to care might be adversely affected, resulting in poor quality. If these factors act as enablers, the overuse of services relative to regional benchmarks could adversely affect health plan financial performance.

Gatekeeping

Gatekeeping is the method for controlling service use. The gatekeeping method derives from the belief that without a knowledgeable clinical expert to organize and control access to care, patients and practitioners will inappropriately use the services. Because patients use services based on second-best information, open access to care results in a lack of conservation about health care resources.

Gatekeepers are practitioners designated by the patient during the health plan enrollment process. The primary care physician designated as gatekeeper coordinates the medical and health care services received by the patient. Often, the gatekeeper uses nurses, nurse practitioners, and physician assistants to assist in providing a wide range of case management services, such as regular checkups, blood pressure monitoring, prescription reorders, and telephone consultation. The emphasis of the gatekeeper and his or her team is to address the patient's primary care needs. The gatekeeping team also controls such services as consultation from specialists, diagnostic testing, hospital admissions, and referral to other delivery systems and sites.

The impact of the gatekeeper team has generally been positive for utilization managers and their organizations. However, physicians and patients have strongly resisted the concept. Physicians generally believe that organizing and coordinating the services and ensuring continuity of care requires excessive time and is not cost-beneficial. In addition, physicians have experienced bureaucratic barriers that have emphasized underuse of services. Finally, patients have resisted the gatekeeper function, believing it to be an intrusion on their right to access medical care. Periodically, news stories report examples of patients denied care because the gatekeepers and utilization review personnel thwarted access to needed services, resulting in adverse clinical outcomes.

Practice Profiling[58,59]

Controlling utilization requires evaluating practice patterns for private practices, hospitals, and health plans. Practice profiling is the collection and analysis of data on practitioner-specific medical practice patterns and the comparison of these data to organizational, professional, or national norms. The objective is to measure the degree of consistency of resource use between individual practitioners and a group of practitioners affiliated with a hospital, health plan, or private practice. Profiling reduces resource consumption, stimulates communication about proper quality of care, and builds knowledge in the organization about the practice patterns of the practitioner group. Feedback from profiling results can initiate dialogue about the rationale for resource consumption, help modify practitioner behavior, and share knowledge about colleagues' practices, as well as identify national and professional "best-practice" benchmarks.

Practice profiling can be used to exclude practitioners from health plan participation. Practitioners who are "statistical outliers" may not have their managed care contracts renewed. Therefore, practice profiling is not a readily accepted procedure. Physicians are concerned that reviews of their practice do not address the quality of the data, create pressure to reduce innovation, and do not take into account the individual characteristics of their patients.[50]

Case Management

Case management is a method that relies on coordinating resources; the efficient use of resources is attained through professional management by an expert coordinator. A case manager controls and monitors the care provided to the patient, making decisions based on in-depth knowledge of the best use of procedures and practitioners. Case managers often consult with primary care physicians and specialists to determine the most appropriate care in the most cost-effective settings. Based on widely available industry standards, patient-focused case management is a useful tool for determining the appropriate level of care. By employing these guidelines, case managers with access to community resources have the ability to place patients in appropriate levels of care, depending on their clinical progress.[49]

The spectrum of case management incorporates the following key elements:

1. Coordinated analysis of diagnostic information
2. Patient education
3. Participative consultation with patients, primary care practitioners, and specialists
4. Participative review of treatment plan options
5. Management of complex cases
6. Management of chronic diseases (disease management)
7. Collaborative decisionmaking regarding treatment
8. Preadmission planning and education
9. Sharing information with families and significant others
10. Readmission prevention
11. Pharmacy management
12. Discharge planning

13. Monitoring of care processes and outcomes
14. Care accountability

Preauthorization[54]

Although overuse of services has been one focus for utilization managers, the additional problem of the wrong use of specialty services or facilities requires review. Preauthorization is the process of assessing the appropriateness of the proposed service or service site; a review opinion either allows the practitioner to proceed with the proposed plan of care or encourages or mandates an alternative approach. Preauthorization places a screen between the practitioner and the subsequent patient service; ideally, alternatives to costly treatments and facilities will emerge. Although physicians view this process as a bureaucratic delay that obstructs the quick response to patient care needs, the medical literature suggests that preauthorization is successful in controlling inappropriate use, such as unnecessary hospital admissions. Finally, patients believe that this increasing stewardship of scarce resources creates an environment of denial of service that impedes the provision of high-quality medical care.

Second Opinions

Second opinion is the process of reviewing a proposed plan of care according to medical necessity. Not only is a second opinion useful for evaluating the provision of specific, noncovered or overused medical procedures, but this process serves as a clinical means for patients, practitioners, and health plan managers to determine whether a proposed treatment plan is clinically correct. Thus, second opinions can be obtained at any point in the patient care process. Second opinions include a clinical re-evaluation of the patient, as well as the treatment choices. They should clarify the benefits, risks, and alternatives of a treatment. Although the second opinion often reinforces the proposed therapeutic plan, the process also introduces discussions about treatment alternatives, thereby enriching the medical care dialogue.

The power of second opinions to control use has been diminished by characteristics of the method. Currently, second opinions have had relatively limited impact on quality of care and cost control because:

1. There is a tendency to support the original opinion
2. Not all patients have access to second opinion sources
3. Conflicting opinions create patient uncertainty
4. Payment for the second opinion is unclear
5. Patients use second opinions as a way to bypass the gatekeeper decisions
6. Patients may file second opinion requests to overturn treatment denial

Discharge Planning

Discharge planning is the process of assisting the patient in leaving a health care facility. Under the best circumstances, discharge planning is instituted at the onset of, or even before, the patient's arrival at the facility. Planning involves estimating the patient's length of stay, expected outcome of clinical care, and the patient's needs at the time of discharge. The utilization manager helps collect and evaluate information, coordinates care and discharge timing, and ensures that required services at the time of discharge do not require an extension of hospital stay.[19]

Disease Prevention and Health Promotion

Utilization management intersects with the field of health prevention and promotion, so resource use can begin before medical care is required. Clearly, utilization managers could reduce hospital admissions if they were able to increase the wellness of the population. From this perspective, health plans, hospitals, or health systems could adopt educational and behavioral strategies that promote healthy living or that prevent the use of acute care, rehabilitation, and long-term care services.

Leading targets of opportunity include:

1. Smoking cessation
2. Weight loss and weight management
3. Exercise promotion
4. General nutrition
5. Immunization promotion
6. Well-baby visits
7. Genetic screening

Utilization Review Studies

Utilization review studies reflect applied research aimed at evaluating under- and overuse of services. These studies are subject to the same rules, constraints, and challenges of traditional applied research and employ a modified scientific method that includes four components:

1. Definitions of the specific utilization review issues
2. Planned interventions
3. Actions to control utilization patterns
4. Impact evaluation

The Process of Utilization Management: Tasks and Stages

Different methods and approaches exist for utilization management. However, when closely examined, many of the required tasks have a common model or purpose and reflect the philosophy of the investigator. Given this uniformity, utilization management studies actually form a continuum of complexity and sophistication. At one end of the continuum are the single case reports, clinical observations, and anecdotes that may not provide conclusive scientific evidence about quality or utilization; at the other end is the randomized, controlled, experimental study with its ability to offer strong proof for the quality or utilization findings. Although not as scientific as a controlled laboratory study—or even a full consensus review by a select and respected scientific panel of experts—the following nine common tasks are fundamental to the study of utilization management.

Task 1: Determine Which Questions Need to Be Answered. Health care organizations are often queried by insiders (boards of directors) and by outsiders (payers and regulators) on the quality of care and the costs of obtaining that quality. The challenge is to identify measures of quality and resource use that reflect the efforts of the health care organization, as well as document aspects of care that are important to patients and purchasers. The first task of utilization management is to determine which questions need to be answered. Questions may arise about current or potential clinical or financial issues, regulatory requirements, or care delivery. In addition, the questions should be correctly asked to ensure that data collected and answers provided are those sought by clinical and administrative leaders.

In some cases, data have already been collected; in others cases, original data must be collected. Data collected to answer questions can be compared to internally or externally developed benchmarks to determine whether improvement is necessary, as well as which areas offer opportunities for improvement. In this way, utilization management contributes to the strategic goals of the organization by providing cost-effective and appropriate services while adhering to the operational goals of the organization by providing timely access to service.

Task 2: Identify Needed Information and Critical Stakeholders. Data are required to answer most questions. Included in this task is the need to identify such factors as the patient populations, diagnoses, treatments, and practitioners of interest; the components of the system that pertain to the problem under study; existing sources of information; and the feasibility of collecting the desired data. Utilization management staff must consider which indicators are relevant to a given project, (e.g., patient satisfaction scores, number of unscheduled returns to surgery, or nosocomial infection rates).[45]

Key stakeholders need to be convinced that the question being asked is important and worth answering. Stakeholders in the clinical process or recipients of care know about the resources necessary for enabling or blocking change.

Many practitioners face the choice of either developing their own data collection systems or buying proprietary programs in which the data to be collected are already specified. Developing in-house information systems programs can be expensive and time-consuming, but proprietary programs may not be flexible enough to adjust to the unique needs of the practitioner.

Task 3: Establish Appropriate Benchmarks. Performance is measured by comparing practitioner outcomes relative to a standard or benchmark. The utilization management program should determine the desired scope and quality of care by establishing benchmarks that, if reached, will indicate satisfactory performance expectations. Benchmarks may address either the process or outcome of health care interventions. Ideally, randomized trials, systematic reviews of the literature, or meta-analyses will have established the validity of a benchmark. However, because evidence of effectiveness is not often available for many interventions, benchmarks often may be identified by expert opinion.[47]

Benchmarks may be established for the structure of care (i.e., does the practitioner have the capacity to provide good care?), the process of care (i.e., is the practitioner delivering necessary and sufficient care?), and the outcomes of care (i.e., are patients realizing the benefits of optimal care?). The benchmarks can be internally or externally generated. External generation may include consensus documents that describe the state of the art. Hospitals may share information that leads to the creation of the group's benchmarks for a wide variety of services. Organizations may also create their own internal benchmarks that can be used to compare individual performance, or the performance of individuals and groups over time. Collecting and sharing benchmarks provides a basis for comparison and can be the foundation for a dialogue among practitioners about common approaches, including the advantages and disadvantages of each.

Task 4: Design, Data Collection, and Data Management Procedures.[59,60] The fourth task is to design the research approach, which consists of identifying the required data and determining how data collection should proceed. Data collection involves several considerations:

1. Designing the research approach (e.g., records review, screening large data sets)
2. Determining the level of inquiry (e.g., individual, team, unit, organization, community)
3. Selecting data sources (e.g., patient records, claims data, patient surveys)
4. Selecting the sample (e.g., to ensure diversity or homogeneity among single practitioners or groups, according to patient severity of illness or demographic distribution)
5. Determining the sampling procedure (e.g., randomly selected records, all records for a given procedure)
6. Determining whether to use both quantitative and qualitative data sources (e.g., claims data in conjunction with physician and staff interviews)

7. Planning for cross-checking to achieve a high level of confidence in results (e.g., searching for agreement among several sources and methods of data)

Task 5: Implement Data Collection and Data Management Procedures. Implementing data collection processes means devoting resources to the task. Personnel may need to be trained or given time to collect data, hardware and software may need to be evaluated or acquired, clinical review criteria will need to be developed or purchased, and policies and procedures need to be documented to provide a standard format for compliance and educational purposes.

Again, practitioners may wish to develop and implement their own data collection and data management procedures, or contract with outside companies for these services. A key question to ask is: Who bears the cost of data collection? Clinical staff might be too busy with clinical services to become research technicians. Utilization staff members might not be able to cover their research data collection needs independently. Although this "hidden" cost of utilization management is distributed to the various service groups, the utilization management team must be held accountable by the system to demonstrate patient care and cost benefits.

Task 6: Evaluate the Data and Present Results. Data must be evaluated and interpreted, preferably using statistical analysis. The data should be compared to the benchmarks to identify any differences or gaps between the care delivered and the benchmark that defines satisfactory care. Organizational issues, such as who looks at the data and what actions they may take based on the results of the data analysis, require scrutiny. A failure in credibility at this point will undermine any interest in using the data for change. In evaluating and presenting the data, utilization management staff is more effective when:

1. Staff members have organizational credibility from other projects
2. Methods and procedures are well explained and competently applied
3. Multiple methods are used to build audience confidence
4. Results are clear, concise, and appropriate to the key questions
5. Results are compared to organizational and to national benchmarks
6. Speculation is labeled as speculation
7. Presentations recognize and involve the audience

Task 7: Develop Guidelines, Policies, and Procedures. The result of utilization research is the development of new policies and procedures that may require change at the individual, unit, or organizational levels. When applying utilization management to prospective or concurrent patient care, the time delay between evaluating the data and implementing new policies and procedures can be especially critical. In any event, if change is to be successful, the four points below need to be addressed:

1. The *rationale, supporting evidence,* and *clarity* of the recommendations for change must be compelling
2. The required *structural* changes, such as adjustments in incentives or work load, need to be widely accepted
3. The *psychology* of change must be managed; many of those affected are reluctant to part with the existing protocol
4. The *management* of the change process, including timelines, continued follow-up, and assigned responsibility for leading and implementing change, must be constant, consistent, and visible

Keep in mind that changes will be better received and acted on if key stakeholders, such as physicians and their clinical teams, are actively engaged in the planning of change.[61]

Task 8: Implement Guidelines, Policies, and Procedures. Guidelines, policies, and procedures must be implemented to actualize system change. Implementation may involve professional and staff awareness and education efforts, new documentation procedures, personnel changes, or equipment purchases. Ideally, these utilization management measures will be integrated with medical quality management measures so that their impact on patient care can be determined. In some cases, the implementation process is rapid; in other cases, changes are better phased in over time.[63,64]

Task 9: Continuously Review the Task List. Under the guidance of a professional utilization manager, the organization should continuously review each task. Because health care systems are dynamic, each change can both eliminate and create problems in the system. The objective is to instill in department members a value and culture of continuous improvement, or "no matter how good our utilization and quality efforts are now, they can always be better." Continuity and follow-up is essential for effective utilization management. The critical aspects for building continuity are:

1. Establishing the belief in accountability for action
2. Establishing the belief that quality and use can be improved in a continuous cycle
3. Establishing a timeframe for periodic review and ensuring that the review process occurs
4. Establishing responsibility for follow-up

Establishing responsibility for follow-up is both a wrap-up of the particular study and a statement about the entire process of utilization and quality management. Ensuring the ongoing nature of the process is the challenge, even in organizations that have done much work in quality and utilization.[62]

Timing of Utilization: Retrospective, Concurrent, Prospective [16,23]

Timing refers to the point during the care process at which utilization review occurs. Three options exist:

1. After the care process has been completed (retrospective)
2. During the care process (concurrent)
3. Before the onset of care (prospective)

Comprehensive utilization management programs often focus on all three stages.

Retrospective Utilization Review is a study of resource use during a particular episode of care and can be performed on an individual basis or by surveying data from many patients. The reviews are frequently based on medical records, or claims and reimbursement data. The effort is designed to test the medical necessity and appropriateness of the care. Pattern analysis is designed to search for clinical routines that regularly lead to unexplained variation in the use of resources. In addition, the data are often compared to national and organizational benchmarks, and feedback is usually given to physicians and clinical teams.[58]

Concurrent Utilization Review is intended to manage resources during the clinical episode. For health plans, attention is paid to length of hospital stay, resources used during the stay, and the depth and breadth of discharge planning. The key issue is timing because data are collected and interventions are made *during the episode of care*, when care can be modified, as opposed to a retrospective review when the lessons can be learned only for the next patient.[65]

Prospective Utilization Review plans for use of services before patient care starts. Thus, preauthorization of services may be required before patients can receive hospital admission, surgery, or other specialty services. Second opinions are a form of prospective utilization review, as they too occur before services are rendered and have the potential to block the provision of what may be defined as unneeded services.

The prospective nature of utilization review indicates an effort to avoid overuse or misuse of services, and this effort is the point of intersection with quality management. Although many utilization managers may be most concerned with the conservation of resources (and thus cost containment), the delay or denial of overuse or misuse of services is actually a quality management question (considering that underuse of needed care puts the patient at risk). Poor quality (over- or misuse) results from inappropriate care. The hunt for wasted resources leads us directly to the quality question.

Information Systems Support

Utilization management programs depend on robust information systems support.[20] Specifically, information systems requirements must support analysis at the five levels of inquiry: individual, team, unit, organization, and community. Some information systems are designed to support analysis on multiple levels, whereas others focus on only individual and organizational metrics.

Regardless of the level of inquiry, information systems must provide data to address several critical questions:

1. What was the type of service and facility where the care was provided?
2. What type of care was provided—diagnostic, therapeutic, acute, or long-term?
3. Who provided the care?
4. How long was the care provided? What was the frequency of contact and follow-up?

These questions should be answered by information systems that provide data for *clinical, administrative,* and *decision support* questions. The basis of clinical information systems is the medical record that provides data on the type, duration, and frequency of care. Administrative systems address the financial and organizational aspects of the care, including new technology development, cost containment, productivity, and return on investment. Decision support is based on clinical and administrative data in support of both strategic and operational decisionmaking.[17,18]

The data-to-action cycle is useful for describing the data management process. Utilization managers follow four steps to convert raw data for use in utilization management:

1. **Data:** raw data regarding cost, quality, and satisfaction for key care processes are gathered
2. **Information:** the data are used to answer clinical and financial questions and to choose opportunities for improvement
3. **Knowledge:** the information is used to study processes in detail, benchmark results, and redesign processes based on best practices
4. **Action:** finally, knowledge is converted to action by publishing results (internally) and using technology to automate processes and provide feedback

The key to this process is that data, information, and knowledge are available at the point of analysis by the utilization management managers or teams.

Measurement Challenges[66]

Several measurement challenges face utilization management leadership, including:

1. Availability and access: data are often not immediately available to utilization management teams

2. Standardization of data and procedures: data and data collection procedures can vary across departmental and organizational boundaries, making comparison with internal and external benchmarks difficult or invalid

3. Data quality: inputs to the information system are flawed, either by error or by varying interpretations of meaning and classification

4. Validity: the data bear only a limited connection to the actual "truth" of the clinical situation (e.g., they are affected by confounding factors, such as variation in severity of illness)

5. Reliability: measurements cannot be repeated without substantial variation in results, calling the original findings into question

6. Multiple data streams: the need to improve validity and reliability by relying on more than one source or procedure for data

7. Timeliness of data delivery: failure of centralized information systems to deliver both standard and specialized requests for data at the time needed by utilization management teams

8. Costs: organizations do not invest sufficient resources in developing the information system infrastructure

Outcomes and Benefits

The outcomes and benefits of utilization management should reflect the level of inquiry whether it involves individual services, team-delivered care, service units, the organization as a whole, or the community.[55,56,57]

A comprehensive utilization management program should classify outcomes and benefits in relation to each level of inquiry.[21] However, some utilization management programs focus on one or more levels of inquiry to the exclusion of others. For example, some hospitals are more concerned with their organizations at the unit, team, and individual levels and are less likely to directly address use of services by the community. Other hospitals believe that examining services by the community is an integral part of their strategic planning and marketing processes.

Regardless of the level of inquiry—from individual to community—there are at least three major outcomes from utilization management:

1. Exposure of the depth and breadth of variation in resource use
2. Consensus on resource requirements
3. Increase in efficiency of resource use

The critical result for administrative leaders is the increase in efficiency of resource use and its implications for cost-reduction. Clinical and administrative leaders regard exposure of the depth and breadth of variation in resource use, and consensus on resource requirements, as the means by which efficiency and cost are addressed.[22]

Finally, expanding our understanding of the contribution of utilization management can be reflected in the long-term benefits to the organization of the review process itself:

1. Recognition as a length-of-stay benchmark performer
2. Determination of multiple areas of savings
3. Elimination of the need for pre-authorization
4. Elimination of the need for notification of admission
5. Elimination of the need for concurrent review

6. Efficient use of personnel
7. Feedback provided by the utilization management group

● Organizational Barriers

Organizational barriers to utilization management efforts present unique challenges for developers of utilization management programs.[68] The following list is representative of these challenges:

1. *Disagreement on the need for transparency.* Many clinical and administrative leaders are unsure of the need for scrutiny of the use of resources. Clinical leaders believe that this is their purview and that their autonomy should not be disturbed. They are unconvinced of the value of reviewing the use of resources during clinical transactions. However, administrative clinical and managerial leaders understand the potential benefits of the retrospective, concurrent, and prospective examination of resource use.

2. *Fear of creeping bureaucracy.* Many clinical professionals, as opposed to administrative leaders, are certain that utilization review is an expansion of the administrative bureaucracy. Regardless of the potential clinical benefits, clinicians believe that they and their staffs will "waste" clinical hours in nonproductive administrative bookkeeping and data manipulation.[25]

3. *Unfocused attention.* Administrative and clinical leaders attempt to evaluate every aspect of clinical operations. Although this evaluation is a desirable goal, successful utilization management programs must focus their efforts on specific targets of opportunity: those procedures or service units that seem to be highly variable in their use of resources and are considered high-volume or high-risk services provided by the organization.

4. *Inadequate resources.* Some utilization management programs develop as pilot experiments. Such programs are often structured on a lean resource base and therefore are inadequately funded. Coupled with ambitious leadership that intended to review all services, this shortage of resources hampers the efforts of utilization management staff. Without sufficient resources, staff will be unable to document contributions to the organization and to the management of patient care within the expected period of time.

5. *Poor team membership.* Utilization management programs have been managed by physicians and nurses. Early efforts did not recognize that strong utilization management programs were interdisciplinary in nature and required a mix of medical service disciplines and administrative department representatives. Although the design of the team membership appears to be a simple task, the participation of various stakeholders becomes a challenge in terms of team characteristics. A balanced group should be composed of junior and senior leaders who possess organizational advocacy and authority.

6. *Excessive untargeted data.* At first, the utilization management program information problem was reflected as a shortage of depth and breadth of data. Many organizations did not have the information systems capability to deliver the required data needed by utilization management teams at their various points of work. However, during the 1990s, the capability of information systems grew rapidly. Presently, utilization management staff can be inundated with reams of data related to the various clinical transactions of the organization. Managing this data overflow is a crucial

problem for utilization management departments because they must ensure that data requests are targeted specifically for the clinical processes under review.

7. *Difficulties in efficiently linking practitioners.* In conjunction with the rapid growth and development of information systems—once the data capability was widely recognized—organizations moved rapidly to ensure that all practitioners were linked to the system. However, utilization management departments faced many problems in efficiently linking practitioners—legacy IT systems, practitioner resistance, new equipment expense, and the archaic start-up processes of information system departments. Unfortunately, the problem of linking practitioners with various organizational privileges and independent group practices remains. To effectively implement utilization management across organizational boundaries, information system capability must cross those boundaries as well.[70]

8. *Legacy measures dominate.* As utilization management staff began developing metrics and benchmarks for review, they were confronted by practitioners and organizational leaders who had pre-existing "favorite measures" that they were comfortable with and reluctant to give up. In some instances, utilization management staff is successful in advocating new and more appropriate measures. However, in other situations, utilization management consists of a hybrid set of current measures as well as outdated legacy measures that might have been in effect since the inception of the organization.

9. *Participation is lacking.* Designers of utilization management programs have recognized that participation by clinicians, employees, and patients is a key program design requirement. However, this design intent is often easier to state than implement. Clinicians, employees, and patients must be convinced that participation in a utilization management program is worth their time. For busy clinical professionals, this process can be an uphill battle. Many program leaders recognize the usefulness of patient participation in the review process, because patients bring a unique perspective to the review of clinical processes, they can describe in anecdotal terms what has occurred within the so-called "smooth clinical process."

10. *Leadership inattention.* Leadership attention to utilization management is essential. Clinicians recognize that their participation in utilization management is of vital interest to the clinical and financial success of the organization. However, they are quick to recognize the absence of the leader. The generation and use of utilization management data requires clinician time and effort at many levels of the organization. The absence of leadership attention to the use of data sends a clear message that the information may not be critical to the clinical and financial success of the organization. Such a message will not "sell" clinician involvement in utilization management.

11. *Failure to achieve demonstrated impact.* Developers of utilization management programs must offer their efforts on "faith." Clinical and administrative leaders can successfully advocate for the start-up and operation of the program. However, after some period of time, the program must demonstrate its contribution to the organization. Just as other clinical units report the outcomes of their clinical efforts and the resulting financial contribution, utilization management leadership must show that the time and energy devoted by clinical staff had an impact (e.g., clinical service improvement, resource conservation, or consensus on procedures and pharmaceutical use). The clinical and administrative staff members will serve as the critical examiners for the presentation of the impact information.

12. *Sustainability over time.* Utilization management departments were started with strong advocacy from the top of the organization and high levels of energy from utilization management staff. These efforts must be sustained over time by demonstrating positive impact and by senior leadership recognition. The contributions of the utilization management effort must be widely disseminated and widely recognized in order to solidify the continued support of clinical and administrative staff at all organizational levels.

Accreditation and Regulatory Oversight Organizations

Several organizations are involved in the development and oversight of the utilization management function. Three organizations are briefly discussed here: Utilization Review Accreditation Commission, the Joint Commission on the Accreditation of Health care Organizations, and the National Committee on Quality Assurance.

Utilization Review Accreditation Commission (URAC)

Established in 1990, URAC (*www.urac.org*) is a nonprofit organization that assists in development of standards for the utilization management programs. Presently, more than 2,000 accreditation certificates have been awarded to 500 health care organizations. The Commission's membership is broad-based, representing a wide range of health care stakeholders, including regulators, employers, consumers, practitioners, information systems specialists, and representatives from the managed care and workmen's compensation fields.

URAC's standards for Utilization management address eight categories:

1. Patient confidentiality
2. Staff qualifications
3. Program qualifications
4. Patient information determinations
5. Review determinations
6. Appeals of determination and certification
7. Expedited review (appeal)
8. Standard appeal

Joint Commission on the Accreditation of Health care Organizations (JCAHO)

Widely recognized for hospital, long-term care facility, and ambulatory care accreditation, JCAHO (*www.jcaho.org*) standards define critical elements for a utilization management program. During accreditation surveys, the presence of utilization management activities serves as a marker of the facility's overall quality-of-care effort. In addition, the JCAHO "Standards on Accreditation—2004" references quality improvement activities that may be included in a utilization management program.

National Committee on Quality Assurance (NCQA)

The NCQA (*www.ncqa.org*) is a nonprofit organization that was founded to address the performance of managed care plans. Accreditation survey efforts are directed to quality improvement and utilization management. The NCQA has incorporated extensive stakeholder participation in developing a comprehensive accreditation process that focuses on:

1. Patient access
2. Provider distribution and mix
3. Provider credentialing
4. Treatment and services
5. Quality management
6. Utilization management
7. Disease management
8. Clinical outcomes
9. Patient satisfaction
10. Appeals and grievances
11. Financial performance

In addition, NCQA has developed the Health Plan Employer Data and Information Set (HEDIS®) reporting system, which has become the standard metric set used by employers and selected government agencies to quantify managed care plan performance. HEDIS® uses 60 metrics divided into 7 categories:

1. Effectiveness of care
2. Access/availability of care
3. Member satisfaction
4. Use of services
5. Cost of care
6. Informed health care choices
7. Health plan descriptive information

Summary

In summary, utilization management is an essential component in a comprehensive program of managed medical services. Performed as part of peer review, administrative review, or public or private agency review, utilization management is a planned and monitored systematic set of programs that encourage both health plan providers and practitioners to meet the health care needs of their patients. When performed in a high-quality and cost-effective manner, utilization management serves as a constructive adjunct for sustaining the medical necessity, appropriateness, and efficiency of the use of health care services. Finally, since utilization management compares the characteristics of specific clinical care to predetermined or established protocols and benchmarks, it is an invaluable tool for supporting disease management, care management, and the evidence-based practice of medicine.

References

1. Carneal G, et al. *The Utilization Management Guide*. Washington, DC: URAC/American Accreditation Health Care Commission; 2000.
2. Griffith FR. *The Well-Managed Healthcare Organization*. Chicago, IL: Health Administration Press; 1995.

3. Donabedian A. Specialization in clinical performance monitoring: What it is and how to achieve it. *Quality Assurance and Utilization Review*. 1990;5(4):114–120.

4. Robinson JC. The end of managed care. *JAMA*. 2001;285(20):2622–2628.

5. Ginsburg PB, Fascino NJ, eds. *The Community Snapshots Project: Capturing Health System Change*. Princeton, NJ: Robert Wood Johnson Foundation; 1995.

6. Kovner AR, Jonas S. *Health Care Delivery in the United States*. New York, NY: Springer Publishing Company; 1999.

7. Wickizer TM, Lessler D, Franklin G. Controlling workers' compensation medical care use and costs through utilization management. *JOEM*. 1999;41(8):625–631.

8. URAC Health Utilization Management Standards, ver 4.2, 2004.

9. Krentz SE, Miller TR. Physician resource profiling enhances utilization management. *Healthcare Financial Management*. 1998;52(10):45–47.

10. Krohn R, Broffman G. Utilization management in a mixed-payment environment. *Healthcare Financial Management*. 1998;52(2):64–67.

11. Lessler DS, Wickizer TM. The impact of utilization management on readmissions among patients with cardiovascular disease. *Health Services Research*. 2000;34(6):1315–1329.

12. Wickizer TM, Lessler D, Boyd-Wickizer J. Effects of health care cost-containment programs on patterns of care and readmissions among children and adolescents. *American Journal of Public Health*. 1999; 89(9):1353–1358.

13. Wolff N, Schlesinger M. Risk, motives, and styles of utilization review: A cross-condition comparison. *Social Science & Medicine*. 1998;47(7):911–926.

14. Cudney A. Increase coordination, effectiveness of case management. *Hospital Case Management*. April 1999: 64–67.

15. Sussman PT. Managing wound care; Utilization management ensures optimal clinical outcomes. *Rehab Management*. April/May 1998:40–131.

16. Spath P. Debate: Retrospective vs. concurrent data collection. *Hospital Peer Review*. May 1999:80–82.

17. Booth BM, Ludke RL, Fisher EM. Inappropriate hospital care and severity of illness: Results from a nationwide study. *American Journal of Medical Quality*. 1998;13(1):36–43.

18. Hornbrook MC, Goodman MJ, Fishman PA, et al. Building health plan databases to risk adjust outcomes and payments. *International Journal for Quality in Health Care*. 1998;10(6):531–538.

19. Brett JL, Bueno M, Royal N, Kendall-Dengin K. Integrating utilization management, discharge planning, and nursing case management into the outcomes manager role. *JONA*. 1997;27(2):37–45.

20. Bowers D. Linking and integrating enterprise-wide health information management data. *Journal of Healthcare Information Management*, 1998;12(3): 81–88.

21. Lippman H. The bottom line on length of stay. *Business and Health*. 2001;19(4):35–38

22. Phillips J.S. Utilization management affects health care practices at Walter Reed Army Medical Center: Analytical methods applied to decrease length of stay and assign appropriate level of care. *Military Medicine*. 1999;164(12):867–874.

23. James B. Implementing practice guidelines through clinical quality improvement. *Frontiers of Health Services Management*. 1993;10(1):3–32.

24. Nelson MF, Christenson RH. The focused review process: a utilization management firm's experience with length of stay guidelines. *Joint Commission Journal on Quality Improvement*. 1995;21(9):477–487.

25. Chassin MR. Is health care ready for six sigma? *Milbank Quarterly*. 1998;76(4):565–587.

26. Cardiff K, Anderson G, Sheps S. Evaluation of a hospital based utilization management program. *Healthcare Management Forum*. 1995;8(1):38–45.

27. Potvin KA, Leclair MC. Comprehensive approach to utilization review based on patient-specific costing data. *Healthcare Management Forum*. 1995;8(4):22–28.

28. Anonymous (from MEDLINE). Patient empowerment touted as next step toward better preventive care. *Disease Management Advisor*. 2001;7(1):1,5–9.

29. Adams KF. Translating heart failure guidelines into clinical practice: Clinical science and the art of medicine. *Current Cardiology Reports*. 2001;3(2):130–135.

30. Atherly A, Culler SD, Becker ER. The role of cost effectiveness analysis in health care evaluation. [Review] [35 refs]. *Quarterly Journal of Nuclear Medicine*. 2000;44(2):112–120.

31. Barnett JR, Coyle P, Kearns RA. Holes in the safety net? Assessing the effects of targeted benefits upon the health care utilization of poor New Zealanders. *Health & Social Care in the Community*. 2000;8(3):159–171.

32. Carneal G, D'Andrea G. Defining the parameters of case management in a managed care setting. *Managed Care Quarterly*. 2001;9(1):55–60.

33. Cooper GS, Armitage KB, Ashar B, et al. Design and implementation of an inpatient disease management program. *The American Journal of Managed Care*. 2000;6(7):793–801.

34. Crim C. Clinical practice guidelines vs actual clinical practice: The asthma paradigm. *Chest*. 2000;118(2 Suppl):62S–64S.

35. Curry SJ. Organizational interventions to encourage guideline implementation. [Review] [25 refs]. *Chest*. 2000;118(2 Suppl):40S–46S.

36. Delnoij D, Van Merode G, Paulus A, Groenewegen P. Does general practitioner gatekeeping curb health care expenditure? *Journal of Health Services & Research Policy*. 2000;5(1):22–26.

37. Donabedian A. A founder of quality assessment encounters a troubled system firsthand. Interview by Fitzhugh Mullan. *Health Affairs*. 2001;20(1):137–141.

38. Donald IP, Jay T, Linsell J, Foy C. Defining the appropriate use of community hospital beds. *The British Journal of General Practice*. 2001;51(463):95–100.

39. Dudley RA, Bowers LV, Luft HS. Reconciling quality measurement with financial risk adjustment in health plans. *Joint Commission Journal on Quality Improvement*. 2000;26(3):137–146.

40. Feldman R. The ability of managed care to control health care costs: How much is enough? *Journal of Health Care Finance*. 2000;26(3):15–25.

41. Glanville I, Schirm V, Wineman NM. Using evidence-based practice for managing clinical outcomes in advanced practice nursing. *Journal of Nursing Care Quality*. 2000;15(1):1–11.

42. Grembowski DE, Diehr P, Novak LC, et al. Measuring the "managedness" and covered benefits of health plans. *Health Services Research*. 2000;35(3):707–734.

43. Habibi KA, Finch SA. Clinicians hold the key to profitable managed care contracting. *Healthcare Financial Management*. 2000;54(7):43–46.

44. Hemingway H, Crook AM, Feder G, et al. Underuse of coronary revascularization procedures in patients considered appropriate candidates for revascularization. *The New England Journal of Medicine*. 2001;344(9):645–654.

45. Hilber DJ, Whitwell KJ, Krumholz DM, Pace CA. The effect of continuous quality improvement on compliance with clinical practice guidelines in an optometric clinic: A retrospective review. *Optometry*. 2000; 71(2):83–90.

46. Jacobson D. Effective strategies for managing pharmacy benefits. *Healthcare Financial Management*. 2001;55(3):41–42.

47. Jencks SF, Cuerdon T, Burwen DR, et al. Quality of medical care delivered to Medicare beneficiaries: A profile at state and national levels. *JAMA*. 2000;284(13):1670–1676.

48. Jennings DL, White-Means SI. Medical care utilization by AFDC recipients under reformed Medicaid. *Journal of Health & Social Policy*. 2001;13(2):21–39.

49. Kalant N, Berlinguet M, Diodati JG, Dragatakis L, Marcotte F. How valid are utilization review tools in assessing appropriate use of acute care beds? *CMAJ*. 2000;162(13):1809–1813.

50. Kerr EA, Mittman BS, Hays RD, Zemencuk JK, Pitts J, Brook RH. Associations between primary care physician satisfaction and self-reported aspects of utilization management. *Health Services Research*. 2000;35(1 Pt 2):333–349.

51. Laditka SB, Laditka JN. Utilization, costs, and access to primary care in fee-for-service and managed care plans. *Journal of Health & Social Policy*. 2001;13(1):21–39.

52. Lawthers AG, McCarthy EP, Davis RB, Peterson LE, Palmer RH, Iezzoni LI. Identification of in-hospital complications from claims data. Is it valid? *Medical Care*. 2000;38(8):785–795.

53. Lessler DS, Wickizer TM. The impact of utilization management on readmissions among patients with cardiovascular disease. *Health Services Research*. 2000;34(6):1315–1329.

54. Liu X, Sturm R, Cuffel BJ. The impact of prior authorization on outpatient utilization in managed behavioral health plans. *Medical Care Research & Review*. 2000;57(2):182–195.

55. Donabedian A. *Explorations in Quality Assessment and Monitoring, Vol. 1*. Health Administration Press. Ann Arbor, MI: 1980.

56. Donabedian A. *The Criteria and Standards of Quality*. Health Administration Press. Ann Arbor, MI: 1982.

57. Donabedian A. Evaluating the Quality of Medical Care. *Milbank Memorial Fund Quarterly*. 1966;44(2):166–206

58. Ritter PL, Stewart AL, Kaymaz H, Sobel DS, Block DA, Lorig KR. Self-reports of health care utilization compared to practitioner records. *Journal of Clinical Epidemiology*. 2001;54(2):136–141.

59. Ross G, Johnson D, Castronova F. Physician profiling decreases inpatient length of stay even with aggressive quality management. *American Journal of Medical Quality*. 2000;15(6):233–240.

60. Rossiter LF, Whitehurst-Cook MY, Small RE, et al. The impact of disease management on outcomes and cost of care: A study of low-income asthma patients. *Inquiry*. 2000;37(2):188–202.

61. Schiff GD, Rucker TD. Beyond structure-process-outcome: Donabedian's seven pillars and eleven buttresses of quality. *The Joint Commission Journal on Quality Improvement*. 2001;27(3):169–174.

62. Shi L, Politzer RM, Regan J, Lewis-Idema D, Falik M. The impact of managed care on the mix of vulnerable populations served by community health centers. *The Journal of Ambulatory Care Management*. 2001;24(1):51–66.

63. Slavin L, Best MA, Neuhauser D. Physician Profiling and Risk Adjustment. *Quality Management in Health Care*. Spring 2000;8(3):78.

64. Tselikis P. Do profiles change the way doctors practice? *Business & Health*. 2000;18(2):23–24.

65. Ubel PA, Baron J, Nash B, Asch DA. Are preferences for equity over efficiency in health care allocation "all or nothing"? *Medical Care*. 2000;38(4):366–373.

66. "The National Health Care Quality Data Set suggests a balance of outcome-validated process measures and condition- or procedure-specific outcome measures. This combination of both process and outcome measures must satisfy the needs of insurers, policy makers, clinicians and consumers." Institute of Medicine, Committee on Quality of Health Care in America. *Envisioning the National Health care Quality Report*, National Academy of Sciences, Washington, DC. 2000:Recommendation 6;p.79.

67. Harris Interactive. Explosive growth of "cyberchondriacs" continues. Available at *www.harrisinteractive.com/harris_poll/index.asp?PID=104*. Accessed August 11, 2000.

68. Griffith JR. Managing the transition to integrated health care organizations. *Frontiers in Health Services Management*. 1996;12(4):4–50

69. Institute of Medicine, Committee on Quality of Health Care in America. *To Err is Human: Building a Safer Health System*. Washington, DC: National Academy of Sciences; 2000:183–184.

70. Duncan KA. Networking healthcare: Community health information systems. *Frontiers of Health Services Management*. Fall 1995;12(1):7,8.

Chapter 3

ORGANIZATION DESIGN AND MANAGEMENT

James T. Ziegenfuss, Jr., PhD

Introduction

The Core Curriculum for Medical Quality Management is organized into six sections. This section is devoted to the relationship between the quality leader and the health/medical organization's design and management. Quality management in health and medical care involves the study of human behavior and attitudes, management systems, and organizational structures that co-produce high quality medical and health care organizations. The field of organization design and management considers how and why people behave as they do in organized settings—hospitals, physician practices, HMOs. Health care quality leaders must be able to address the following organization and management issues in quality improvement, presented here as five questions:

1. Why has the field moved beyond clinical quality assurance?
2. What does systems thinking contribute to quality management?
3. What are the critical responsibilities and competencies of a quality management leader?
4. What roles does the quality leader play (with what authority and power)?
5. What are the critical skills of quality management leadership (planning, teams, strategy formulation, evaluation, and feedback)?

This chapter briefly addresses each of these questions.

The challenge for quality management leaders is to design organizational structure and management systems that lead to open assessments of the current state of quality, continuous efforts to improve quality, and ongoing monitoring of quality of care. By providing knowledge of how and why individuals and groups behave as they do, organization behavior theory and concepts help quality leaders to design management systems that enable physicians and support staff to attain and maintain high medical quality through management and organizational leadership.

Quality management leaders are knowledgeable about "individual level" issues such as perception, motivation, and satisfaction as well as group dynamics,

95

characteristics of high-performance teams, and intergroup collaboration strategies. Effective quality leaders know how the diverse elements of organization design contribute to high quality organizations. These elements include incentives and reinforcement strategies, strategic planning, development and maintenance of culture and values, and the psychological aspects of open access to information and data feedback. The underlying premise of organization and management study is that medical care is provided in an organizational context, a context that can enhance and support quality, or undercut the work of clinical teams. Quality leaders are expected to contribute to the organization's strategic leadership, in roles such as advocates and design experts. We have been developing this view over the past several decades. This evolution is the groundwork of our current organizational systems viewpoint

Near-Term History

In the 1980s and 1990s, medical quality professionals and researchers examined the contributions of industrial quality improvement, led by Crosby,[1] Deming,[2] and Juran,[3] to see whether they could address the deficiencies of traditional quality assurance and the complexities and incompleteness of assessment without improvement. For example, McLaughlin and Kaluzny[4] saw the move to total quality management as a paradigm shift to a whole new way of thinking about the philosophy, research, and practice of quality.[4] What they meant by "paradigm shift" is explained in three summary points: (1) the concept of quality was broadened beyond clinical to organization, and beyond assurance and assessment to improvement; (2) new approaches—total quality management (TQM) and continuous quality improvement (CQI)—are now tested empirically; and (3) refinements in TQM occur over a period of years until it becomes the prevailing paradigm. The traditional professional model—clinical leaders having authority and responsibility—that guided quality assurance efforts shifted toward a total quality management model that put executives in leadership roles. The subject became the "whole organization" including and now going beyond clinical transactions.

According to McLaughlin and Kaluzny,[4] traditional quality assurance was characterized by the individual responsibility of professionals who maintained autonomy and both administrative and professional authority over quality. Quality assurance teams established goals through planning. Many of the goals were driven by responses to complaints. Goal attainment failure was indicated by retrospective performance review.

In contrast, the total quality management (TQM) model for quality assurance offers a collective, management-led, team-oriented approach.[4] The model features interdisciplinary teams, wide participation, flexible planning, benchmarking inside and outside the industry, and an orientation toward continuous improvement in every aspect of medical care.

How is this different from traditional quality assurance approaches? Planning is flexible and progress is noted by benchmarks that are periodic and concurrent. Continuous improvement of all key activities is the goal. Data are shared and medical executives and boards are more intimately involved.

The shift from the quality assurance approach of the 1970s and 1980s—an approach that has been described as a "provider-oriented, defensive response to requirements of external agencies"—was a dramatic one. "Whole organization" quality management is proactive and internally driven—a continuous seeking of the best clinical and administrative structure, which requires attention to design and redesign of services and organizations. For some organization scientists, such as Ackoff,[5,6] quality is a characteristic of a desirable future—an idealized point to be strived for through continuous improvement. Berwick thinks of this as changing "mental models" regarding how we think about quality improvement.[7]

As a critical representative of this shift in thinking,[8] Berwick et al. outlined the basic principles of quality management that support the total organization approach now prevalent.

1. Productive work is accomplished through processes.
2. Sound customer-supplier relationships are absolutely necessary for sound quality management.
3. The main source of quality defects is problems in the process.
4. Poor quality is costly.
5. Understanding the variability of processes is a key to improving quality.
6. Quality control should focus on the most vital process.
7. The modern approach to quality is thoroughly grounded in scientific and statistical thinking.
8. Total employee involvement is critical.
9. New organizational structures can help to achieve quality improvement.
10. Quality management employs three basic, closely integrated activities: quality planning, quality control, and quality improvement.

Clearly, the total quality management approach is not a "one-clinician-is-the-problem" perspective. The necessary analysis and set of responses actually involve a full review of the organizational context of individual action (including the financial impact).[1] As noted in many of the principles, thinking in terms of service delivery process and systems is crucial. The Berwick principles are increasingly found in the quality improvement efforts of hospitals, HMOs, and group practices, as well as of individual units and departments. In 1993, Juran saw this as a renaissance,[9] a return to interest in the quality journey.

Quality improvement activities in health care today:

- represent a change in philosophy from individual and unit to organizational, and from reactive/punitive to proactive/developmental
- borrow strategies and methods from the industrial sector
- offer strong case experience and growing research and development in both health care and other industries
- are truly trans- and interdisciplinary in nature
- have external regulatory support
- offer assistance in competitive situations
- are costly and still relatively underutilized

What is the quality leader's contribution to this effort? The focus in this chapter will be on the following eight areas, judged to be critical to understanding the quality leader's success:

- Organizational systems thinking
- Responsibilities and competencies
- Roles, authority, and power
- Planning and vision
- Group dynamics
- Strategy formulation and implementation

- Evaluation
- Feedback

This group of elements is certainly not exhaustive, but it does include the key areas of knowledge and skill needed by quality management leaders in their unique and important task.

Organizational Systems Thinking

We have shifted how we think about the work of the quality management leader. Instead of monitoring only clinical transactions—often individual episodes between doctors and patients—quality leaders are now expected to attend to the "whole organization"—from resources to strategy to executive decisionmaking. The target of the quality leader's attention is the "organized social system" in which medical care is produced and delivered. Leaders must know more about this target in order to effectively maintain and improve its capabilities. Organization theory is the usual label.

At the start of the 21st century, theorists view the organization as a whole, which is guided by values and principles, interacting subsystems, and structures and processes of integration. A complex web of interlocking systems—both social and technical in nature—these systems include the medical task and core medical technology, the skills and abilities of clinical teams and administrators needed to complete the work, and the individual and group behaviors that comprise a social system. The quality management leader uses "system thinking" to coordinate these diverse systems to assess, improve, and control quality using organization theory and behavior as a base.[10]

A definition of systems is in order. One of the most straightforward is by Ackoff:

A system is a set of two or more elements that satisfies the following three conditions: (1) The behavior of each element has an effect on the behavior of the whole. (2) The behavior of the elements and their effects on the whole are interdependent. (3) However subgroups of the elements are formed, each has an effect on the behavior of the whole and none has an independent effect on it.[6 (p 15)]

As systems thinkers, physician leaders recognize that medical quality is impacted by incentives, team behavior, and cultural values that support open review of quality data.

Clinical and administrative managers direct and lead the quality initiative based on a belief that organizations are "sociotechnical systems." The quality management task is sociotechnical, which means that medical/clinical technology and procedures—as well as individual and group psychology—are a part of the challenge. Pasmore explained this view by highlighting several key assumptions.[11] A sociotechnical view of quality improvement means that:

- quality derives from addressing whole jobs, not parts of jobs.
- workers must have autonomy to improve quality.
- authority for quality improvement must be delegated.
- group rewards must support team-based quality improvement.
- barriers to quality improvement must be eliminated.
- quality improvement evolves by recognizing the value of people,
- innovation for improvement supports quality.
- quality is driven by internal and external factors.

Deming has long emphasized that quality improvement is both a social and technical task: "improvement of the (manufacturing) process includes better allocation of human effort . . . It means removal of barriers to pride of workmanship both for production workers and for management and engineers."[2 (p 51)] This call to address the way we work was heard. "Fix the process"—already noted by others—became a call to action.[12] This involves a redesign of the medical production and delivery system process. "Improve constantly and forever the system of production and service"[2 (p 49)]. Technical design—new therapies and procedures—must continue to move forward. This technological imperative in medicine and health care ensures a need for the technical review of quality.

A psychosocial dimension also exists. What about the cultures and psychology of hospitals and HMOs? "People must be secure about their jobs in the future, and must know that acquisition of new skills will facilitate security."[2 (p 203)] This social dimension also is a co-producer of quality, with modern models linking both perspectives. We will consider one example.

Kast and Rosenzweig's thirty-year-old conception of the organization is consistent with current sociotechnical thinking now accepted in the field. They view the organization as open to the environment (i.e., outside the institution events, and policy changes are recognized and planned for) and as composed of a number of subsystems under the following five titles:[13]

1. The product and technical subsystem (e.g., clinical services)
2. The structural subsystem (e.g., incentives)
3. The psychosocial subsystem (e.g., satisfaction, team behavior)
4. The managerial subsystem (e.g., leadership)
5. The culture, goals, and values subsystem (e.g., climate, shared assumptions)

To understand the organization and management aspects of quality, this mental model is the underpinning—the *architectural target* for design, development, and change.[14] It is necessary to describe briefly the nature of each of these subsystems, which are the targets of quality improvement work. The following descriptions are based on Kast and Rosenzweig's original work, adapted with the research and thinking of other theorists:[15]

1. The *product and technical subsystem* refers to the knowledge required to design, develop, and distribute patient care services. The product and technical subsystem includes the "core work" of the health care organizations—teaching and providing medical care. The product/technical system develops as a result of the task requirements of the organization, and varies depending on the particular activities of the organization as a whole and of its subunits, such as departments. The technology used in hospitals differs significantly from that used in an HMO. The products and technology of a hospital emergency room are different from those in a laboratory. The product/technology subsystem is shaped by the production and delivery process, specialization of knowledge and skills required, types of equipment involved, and layout of facilities.

2. The *structural subsystem* involves the ways in which the tasks of the organization are divided (differentiation) and coordinated (integration). Organization charts, position and job descriptions, and rules and procedures define the structure in a "formal sense." Structure is also defined by emergent and formal patterns of authority, communication, and workflow. The organization's structure is the basis for establishing formal relationships between the clinical production process and worker psychology. For example, financial incentives are a structural tool that can be used to enhance the quality of clinical performance.[16] Many examples of flawed performance are found to be encouraged by wrong-headed reward systems that provide structural support for undesired

behaviors.[17] Informal interactions and relationships link the technical and psychosocial subsystems and can bypass the formal structure.

3. Every organization has a *psychosocial subsystem*—the psychosocial dynamics of individuals and groups that interact. Forces outside the organization, and internal characteristics such as technology and structure, help to establish the organization's psychological climate within which physicians, administrators and staff perform their clinical and administrative roles and activities. Subsystem elements may include individual behavior and motivation, status and role relationships, and group dynamics, as well as the values, attitude, expectations, and aspirations of the people in the organization. For example, some believe participatory involvement is central to continuous improvement.[18] As a result of this unique mix, the psychological climate differs significantly from organization to organization. Certainly, the climate in which an HMO claims staffer works is different from that of the nurse on a pediatric unit, or a doctor in emergency surgery. Psychosocial aspects of organizations are both shaped and supported by management.

4. The *managerial subsystem* is the integrator that relates the organization to its environment; sets the goals; develops comprehensive, strategic, and operational plans; designs the structure; and establishes evaluation and control processes. Managerial activities have traditionally been described in terms of planning, organizing, developing, directing/leading, and controlling. These duties are performed through a series of management roles—interpersonal, informational, and decisional.[19] More recently, design, education, and stewardship have been viewed as core duties.[20] Thus the managerial task includes curriculum development[21] and the training of new medical leaders.[22] Management coordinates and integrates the production, structural, psychosocial, and cultural subsystems.

5. *Organizational culture* is the last of the five subsystems. To be successful and to survive, organizations must meet social requirements, which comprise the goals and values of the external environment. Here we include the concept of corporate culture[23,24] and the ability to understand culture as part of clinical and administrative problem-solving.[25] This subsystem links the goals and values of the members of the organization with those of the broader society.

Each of these subsystems is a part of the architecture that must be created to stimulate quality improvement, yet each contains barriers such as inadequate clinical knowledge, poor teamwork, and resistant leadership.[26,27] They are considered "internal" to this perspective of the organization (i.e., hospitals, private practice, HMO). There is an "external suprasystem," which includes all forces outside the "boundaries" of the organization (defined by the five systems). These forces can include a diversity of issues such as national and international trends, climatic and competitive situations (some of which are barriers to quality).[28] A sample of the rich mix of these external aspects includes the following categories of environmental content:

- Economics (e.g., state and natural economy)
- Politics (e.g., cost containment, policy initiatives)
- Technology (e.g., new equipment, pharmaceuticals)
- Social and demographics (e.g., single family, aging, crime)
- Law (e.g., malpractice)
- Culture (e.g., expectations, alternative medicine)
- Natural resources (e.g., water, weather)
- Globalization (e.g., war, pollution)

Additional categories of environmental content, such as communications and transportation, could be added; all can potentially affect medical quality from "outside" the organization—hospital, private practice, HMO. They present both opportunities for progress and demonstrations of wasted resources.[29]

Is there connectedness between Deming's approach to quality and systems thinking? Dyer cites Banathy's work[30] as part of the effort to define systems thinking with these characteristics: guiding vision and core values, group-led design, environment inclusion, design as an evolutionary process, and promotion of a new design culture. This view of quality management—incorporating Deming's philosophy and approach—fits quite well with these requirements and with Ackoff's basic definition of systems thinking.

With this perspective, every quality management problem is potentially a five-system problem—from technical clinical issues to attitudes to executive behavior. This approach to improvement both evolves from and reinforces our understanding of organizational thinking. Early views of medical failures and quality improvement approaches emphasized the clinical—technical. The human relationists and behavioral scientists advocated the importance of the psychology and sociology of clinical teams that focused on motivation, group dynamics, and related people-oriented factors. The systems school (multiple subsystems) concentrated on methods of integration and linkage processes. Each approach to quality improvement emphasized a particular subsystem, with little recognition of the others. Today we think in multi-system terms. Quality management leaders must think not just about medical procedure but about structural incentives, teamwork, strategy, and core values. In short, they must act as systems thinkers to effectively solve quality problems.[31,15]

Responsibilities and Competencies

What, then, are the leadership requirements for quality leaders? In 1986, Delbecq listed the behaviors that he felt defined leadership: visioning, communication, focus on people, enduring, and managing innovation.[32] Linking these to our quality improvement task illustrates the behaviors that physician executives and quality managers must exhibit in order to help the organization move toward higher quality on the board level, the senior management level, and the unit level. Here we focus first on the specification of the future, a higher quality future.

Leaders, who provide a clear sense of direction, must engage in a process of envisioning quality. For quality improvement, this means that leaders direct the organization toward a higher level of quality through a co-produced and communicated vision. An executive team might jointly describe a vision in this manner: "Our hospital will be among the lowest in complications, unexpected mortalities, infections, and accidents of all types. We will work to provide the clinical teams with the highest quality support—sufficiently high enough that they recognize it. And we will ensure that the patients, board, staff, and community know of this commitment and accomplishment."

Planning is required to improve quality; as Juran noted, quality is planned. A health care organization's strategic and operational plans should include goals for quality improvement. Physician leaders must take action to improve quality, including the acquisition of appropriate new and replacement equipment and the development of such quality improvement tools as information systems and team processes. Physicians show leadership by talking about quality issues, by balancing cost pressures and quality needs, and by spreading the quality message inside and outside the organization. Finally, physician leaders use a quality control system for both clinical and administrative work, initiating and supporting clinical and organizational quality improvement. A vision of quality with enough detail to monitor its fulfillment (benchmarks) demonstrates executive leadership.

Executives and managers communicate their concern for and desire to improve quality. "A leader assures integrity and celebrates achievements." Physician leaders inform management and clinical personnel of the importance of quality, and of both quality successes and quality failures. The rites and symbols of public events communicate the concern and the vision. Clinical executives and clinical managers demonstrate the value of quality in the organization by using awards and rewards—public recognition for personnel who engage in quality improvement and who provide high-quality services. And when unpleasant incidents occur, they are recognized as present opportunities for leadership. Quality is either enhanced through intervention or very subtly sabotaged by looking the other way. True leaders of quality improvement are more than just managers of the production process. Leaders are more heavily invested than managers in:

- Critical decisionmaking
- Strategic decisions
- Option widening
- Opportunistic surveillance
- Goal setting and changing
- Being proactive

Leaders who are concerned with quality intervene, whereas managers may tend to smooth over the problem. Of course the quality leader's job is a complex mixture of roles and responsibilities.

New quality management leaders rarely have a keen sense of what it is they will be expected to do. With the notion that they lead their organization's quality effort, five responsibilities are essential: (1) internal advocacy and spokesmanship; (2) policy, planning and vision; (3) delivery-system-decision support; (4) analysis and control of quality; and (5) external liaison and representation.[33] These five areas become manifested in the well known managerial competencies of: industry knowledge, vision and development skills, communication and interpersonal ability, which are reflected in the following tasks and activities (other duties may be added to this set, but it seems that these are fundamental):

1. *Internal advocacy and spokesmanship.* The medical quality leader takes the lead in articulating and stimulating discussion of quality values with clinical and administrative staff. The philosophy and purpose of quality in the institution—hospital, private practice, HMO—is talked about and advocated in many forums, from administrative meetings to departmental specialty conferences. The quality leader is expected to be able to diplomatically raise the "quality flag," which promotes patient services, professionalism, and corporate success.

2. *Policy, planning, and visioning.* How well is the quality perspective represented in strategic discussions? Does it rate the prominence given to cost reduction, profit margins, and market share? Here the leader is expected to identify and present the competitive advantages of quality and—most importantly—to lead the development of the organization's formal policies on quality management. Quality policy design includes consideration of objectives, quality management methods, resources, staffing, and impact. And, as an extension of this effort, we look to the leader for help in creating a vision of the quality future.

3. *Delivery system decision support.* Most health and medical care organizations are considering redesign of their delivery systems. Some are developing greater internal integration of departments and more sophisticated information systems to track patients, services, and financial transactions. Others are involved in discussions about mergers and acquisitions. Pushing integration, quality leaders "must be able to jump into complex situations quickly, relate to many levels of authority smoothly and bridge gaps in culture and perception."[34] Every organization faces both daily operating problems and the need for continuous change. Embedded in the critical point of analysis is redesign and re-engineering efforts.

4. *Analysis and control of quality.* Within the existing system there is an ongoing need to identify and collect quality data, conduct the required analyses, and act on the results to stimulate continuous improvement of the delivery system. The quality leader is expected to coordinate team processes such as deciding which information is relevant and managing the data feedback. The leader must understand the technical tools of quality management *and* the social psychology of group and intergroup change because the task is sociotechnical in nature.

5. *External liaison and representation.* Purchasers, regulators, and consumers now seek information on quality of care. We expect the chief executive to be the quality leader in a symbolic sense, establishing a culture with quality values and a continuous improvement philosophy. We expect the medical quality leader to fully represent those values in practice, helping the organization to meet and exceed professional and accreditation standards. When industry purchasers and oversight groups request data, examples of continuous improvement gains, and detailed descriptions of quality management practice, someone must respond; the medical quality leader assumes the leadership and coordinating responsibility.

The work required of the quality leader is both significant and extensive. In a period of enormous cost pressures, much change, and considerable anxiety about the policy impact on patient care, this role is vital. And, as we think about the requirements of the role we can quickly see its complexity: a set of roles acted out by quality leaders.

Roles, Authority, and Power

To fulfill the responsibilities presented above, quality management leaders act in several key roles in the quality system. First, quality leaders must be *technical experts* guiding the institution—hospital, private practice, HMO—to a clear and effective system based on state-of-the-art quality philosophy and methods. The quality leader must know the technology of the quality management field (Donabedian's concept of the clinical performance specialist). Second, they must act as *educators*, teaching clinical and administrative staff about the primary and advanced knowledge and skills that have developed in the quality field. The quality leader must spend time explaining why and how quality management contributes to the institution's objectives. Third, they must act as process *experts*, using interpersonal communication and group skills to lead both management and clinical personnel through the development and usage of a system of quality management. The quality leader must utilize interpersonal and communication skills when working with individuals and groups. Finally, quality leaders must be able and willing to act as *evaluators*, constantly assessing the state of their quality management system and searching for ways to improve its design and operations. Quality leaders must help the institution develop as well as help members make informed decisions.

The roles of the quality leader are further illustrated by using Henry Mintzberg's classic set of managerial roles.[19] Think of the quality leader as the manager of the quality process in its entirety. (See Table 3–1).

Successful performance in these roles requires that quality leaders have the authority and power to influence behavior (i.e., to create concerted, coordinated efforts to deliver and constantly improve quality).

What authority do quality specialists have, and what sources of power do they use to change quality levels? First, successful quality specialists use *charismatic authority*, derived from personal characteristics such as warmth, sensitivity, strength, and firmness. They also use *professional authority*, derived from their reputation in their specific professional area (i.e., medical specialty) and from professional recognition received throughout their careers. Quality specialists rely on *traditional authority* (history of program support) if the quality specialist position has become a tradition. Many also use *rational legal authority*, which focuses on law, official rules and procedures, and professional standards. Quality leaders most often use charismatic and professional authority; they come from an already established profession such as medicine or nursing and they have been chosen as a quality specialist because of their technical and social skills (i.e., individual and group relations).

The power base that supports quality specialists' change efforts has several different dimensions. The quality specialist can rely on both the *reward* and the *coercion* dimensions of power; without resolution of medical problems and complaints, rewards may not be given to individuals and departments. There is a *referent* dimension to the quality specialist's power, based on the formal and informal relation to the senior manager (i.e., CEO or medical staff chief) supporting the quality im-

Table 3–1   Management Roles and Functions in Quality Improvement

Management Roles	Management Functions in Roles
Interpersonal Roles	
• Figurehead	To lead quality planning
• Leader	To direct and lead organization-wide quality effort
• Liaison	To communicate up to board, down to departments and quality teams, and outside to environment
Informational Roles	
• Monitor	Of quality progress
• Disseminator	Of quality improvement ideas and successes
• Spokesperson	For internal and external quality efforts
Decisional Roles	
• Entrepreneur	To initiate new and innovative CQI strategies, methods
• Disturbance handler	To resolve quality-generated conflicts within and between teams, departments, etc.
• Resource allocator	To distribute/develop resources for quality improvement
• Negotiator	To settle on quality requirements, internal and external

Source: Adapted from Henry Mintzberg, *The Manager's Job: Folklore and Fact.* Harvard Business Review, 1975.

provement process. Quality specialists also rely on their *problem-solving expertise* and *personal abilities* as aspects of their power base; power flows to quality specialists as a result of their technical ability and problem-solving performance. Over time, the quality specialist's authority becomes *legitimate* because it is recognized by the organization.

The roles of the quality specialist and his or her authority and power base must be fitted to the approach to quality whether it involves traditional clinical quality assurance or the systems-oriented organizational path. The punitive policing approach of the 1960s and 1970s did not call for the helping/consultation mode; the quality assurance specialist in that era pointed blame and punished. The "whole organization" model moves the quality specialist beyond the clinical performance role that characterizes some quality specialist descriptions.

Planning and Vision

As medical quality leader in the institution, planning the quality future is a core responsibility. The quality leader will have the ability to design and implement a planning process involving at least these four steps: (1) an external analysis of threats to quality (e.g., market forces) and of opportunities for improvement outside the boundaries of the organization; (2) an analysis of internal structures and their contribution to quality; (3) development of a vision of the desired quality future; and (4) identification of key strategies and actions that will move the organization from its *quality present* to its *desired quality future*. The leader must ensure that quality is the mission[35] and that there are measures and guideposts to enable the organization to assess progress in quality improvement along the way. Planning is both long term and short term, with activities in each timeframe making a contribution to future quality.

Quality management policy and planning now include a wide range of philosophies and techniques. Medical quality leaders must stop to consider the respective contributions of the emerging approaches. Advocates of the various models of planning and future design are competing to define *the one best approach*. But each has a place in the quality management repertoire because they all contribute to clinical and administrative system redesign and, ultimately, to improvement to patient services. Consider this view of the relationships among three popular models of planning and redesign: continuous clinical quality improvement, re-engineering, and visioning all must be familiar to medical quality leaders.[36]

Continuous quality improvement can generally be viewed as the never-ending search for improvement in medical procedures and outcomes. In practice, the work uses a diagnosis-planning-action-evaluation cycle based on data collection and analysis to effect continuous incremental improvement to existing practice. For example, with the coronary artery bypass procedure, we have attained lower infection rates, quicker procedures with decreasing lengths of hospital stay, and even increasingly conservative use of the technique.

Re-engineering is a radical and dramatic change in an existing process, resulting in a "leap" forward in approach and practice. Used for restructuring and for cost improvements,[37] it is now being tested in the private and public sectors.[38] Consider the coronary artery bypass example used in the preceding paragraph. Although we could argue about the "degree of leap," the use of stents to prop open arteries may be one example of re-engineering. Another more dramatic example is the emerging use of small-incision procedures. In these process redesigns, we are attempting to address the "bypass challenge" in a significantly different way.

But with both continuous improvement and re-engineering strategies underlying assumptions and problems may not be addressed.

> It is a mistake to suppose that efficient production of product and service can with certainty keep an organization solvent and ahead of the competition. It is possible and in fact fairly easy for an organization to go downhill and out of business making the wrong product or offering the wrong type of service, even though everyone in the organization performs with devotion, employing statistical methods and every other aid that can boost efficiency.[2] (pp 25–26)

Visioning involves the creation of a desired quality future that may imply continuous improvement to existing practices, radical changes, new process approaches, and a reformulating of the conditions that created the problem in the first place. It requires not just revised clinical practice but also the building of core values, or "corporate character."[39,40] Let us revisit the coronary artery bypass example.

Along with continuously improved current procedures and radically new approaches to completing a coronary artery bypass, we could vision a community-wide effort to reduce the incidence and prevalence of heart disease (e.g., the healthy communities movement). In addition to reactive treatment of disease, we incorporate planned redesign of causative conditions. This approach takes a whole systems perspective in the sense that we recognize the contributing factors such as: missing information and education, patient behaviors of low exercise and poor eating habits, and peer and public support of the current causes of the problem. Nutrition, exercise, smoking, and other wellness issues are addressed along with acute care treatments in an attempt to create a vision of "greater heart-health future." As Juran has noted, poor quality does not happen by accident—it is designed. Given our present behaviors, poor quality of health is designed to be a part of our personal and community future, but this does not need to be the case. Incremental and radical process improvement in treatment can be accompanied by "stretch goals" of significantly improved population health (i.e., pushing quality beyond the institution's walls).

When we think of planning quality management in an inclusive way, we mean both interventions (such as continuous quality improvement and re-engineering) and preventive integrated actions (such as new visions). The vision enables us to describe and purposely design our most desired future. Quality management leaders have already found that it is not a matter of one approach or the other; all three are part of a package of planning and development tools used to improve quality of care for patients. The visioning process can be used at any level of the system, from service to department to institution to country.[41]

For quality leaders, the visioning task has taken on increasing importance and is therefore due some additional comment regarding the basic components. Using traditional clinical quality assurance thinking, the vision would include clinical, education, and prevention services directly related to patient care. With a sociotechnical organization systems perspective, the scope of the vision is greatly enlarged to include both traditional clinical changes and new technologies such as the Internet.[42]

A visioning procedure includes eight tasks, regardless of the level of the organization. Ackoff describes his process as follows:

> Design is a cumulative process. It is usually initiated by using a very broad brush. Therefore, the first version is a rough sketch, then details are gradually added and revisions are made. The process continues until a sufficiently detailed design is obtained to enable others to carry it out as intended by its designers.[6] (pp 113,114)

Summarizing the approaches and procedures of many experts leads up to these eight general steps:

1. Develop a generalized vision of a desired quality future that is exciting and challenging to clinical, support, and administrative staff (this applies to the whole organization).
2. Describe the dominant quality goals and values of the future—practice, unit, or organization (the culture of quality).
3. Describe the expected quality levels of clinical care from surgery to nursing services to ancillary support (classical clinical quality parameters).
4. Redesign the structure to enhance the quality of clinical and administrative services, including satisfaction and effectiveness (structural design and incentives).
5. Describe the desired psychosocial climate in the future, from expectations to satisfaction levels to group dynamics (psychological attitudes and commitment to continuous improvement).
6. Describe desired quality-enhancing management behaviors, from planning to development to control (leadership).
7. Develop an integrated vision of the newly designed unit or organization.
8. Regularly evaluate progress toward the desired quality future.

Completing these tasks leads to a vision of the quality future that is both comprehensive and detailed. This sequence ensures that the creative process begins with a vision of the quality of the whole unit, department, or organization, but it also forces the quality team to address specific design needs of individual organization subsystems and parts, from medical processes to management control (the architecture of quality). The result is a "designed quality future" that is derived from both a broad vision and from the specific operational changes that need to be made to achieve the quality future.

Quality leaders have long been accustomed to seeking technical and clinical improvements. Planning also attacks psychological barriers, because we find frequently that "the principle obstruction between us and the future we most desire is ourselves."[6 (p 123)] The path to higher quality is blocked by people, purposely or inadvertently, through poor delivery systems design and a psychological belief that the current system is good enough. There are six behavioral benefits of quality planning (parallel to Ackoff's contributions of idealized design):

1. *Participation* in quality improvement is increased at all levels.
2. *Aesthetics* and *values* can be injected into the quality debate.
3. *Consensus* is created around quality diagnoses and required actions.
4. *Commitment* to continuous development is generated.
5. *Creativity* is encouraged and enhanced.
6. *Implementability* of quality improvement solutions is expanded.

There are clear connections between Ackoff's points of participation, values, and commitment, and Deming and Crosby's principles. The themes of people, philosophy, and collaboration, which resound in works by total quality management proponents Deming and Crosby, are also the themes that Ackoff stresses in his design process for corporate futures.

Most visions—if not all—depend on the participation and support of clinical and administrative groups. In short, quality is a "group activity." Teams are fundamental aspects of quality management.

Group Dynamics

Quality management leaders know that group effectiveness is one critical element of the design and operation of quality maintenance and improvement. Partnerships with physicians, administrators, staff, and patients are required.[43] Leaders understand and act on the fundamental elements of effective groups, including scope and purpose, structure, time management, participation strategies, conflict management, action focus, and impact assessment (the "quality" of the group process). Many clinical staff members complain quite rightfully that meetings are wasted time that has little impact on the clinical or administrative work of the institution. They complain about poor group, team, and committee management skills. Integrating administrative and clinical agendas, managing diverse power and authority levels, and ensuring focused attention to the quality improvement objective requires experience and training in both small- and large-group management. Building a team is a core task in medicine, manufacturing, and sports.[44]

Many, if not most, quality leaders work with a committee. Using the group to foster quality improvement requires the leader to attend to the design and functioning of the group, recognizing the synergy between participative quality management and shared governance.[45] Many quality management groups are now well developed, with experienced members, funding, and professional leadership. Some are extremely effective in representing their various constituencies—patients, clinicians, managers, and regulators. Their power to generate continuous improvement is both *persuasive* and *coercive*. Once engaged, clinical and administrative members find participation to be both rewarding and effective in attacking quality-of-care issues about which they are deeply concerned. The literature on medical quality devoted specifically to the role and functioning of quality management groups is somewhat thin; however, significant work on group performance in general has been done. Groups developed to perform health care quality management are more likely to function at a high level if the following conditions are met:[46]

1. *Size and structure.* The preferred committee size is 8–15, not the "convention" size of 25 dictated by some representation-oriented institutions. The difficulty is that many disciplines and functions want a "seat at the table"; but with too many participants, there is literally not enough "air time." A simple and lean structure is desired and not easily maintained because even small groups can quickly become bureaucratic. Extensive minutes, subcommittees, and ad hoc groups may seem useful in addressing specific topics, but they add complexity that undercuts flexible and speedy movement.

2. *Shared vision.* Coproduced by leaders and the group, the members have a clear sense of where they are going (i.e., the quality-improved future) and how the committee's work fits into the institution's objectives. This vision is not pre-formed but is worked out with the group.

3. *Focused objectives.* Specific near-term projects are clearly defined. Members' work is focused on several top-priority projects. Members have chosen objectives that are manageable within the timeframe and resources, and a defined purpose that is limited in scope. Do we collectively understand our group's primary objectives and tasks for this defined period? The more focused this charge, the more effective the group's output will be. Targeted and focused creativity means leaders keep to the core topic, pushing ideas that further discussion, open new options, or lead to specific actions. These are all channeled toward the group's primary mission.

4. *Leadership.* The leader of the group attends to both the task—quality improvement—and to the relationship between the members. The leader knows that over time, the power of the team will

add significant value to the task only if attention is paid to team management. Groups require informed, participative leadership that is determined to receive input from all members. Members rapidly come to understand the style and orientation of the leader. At the early meetings, input may or may not be solicited and respected, decisions may or may not be consensus driven, and meeting agendas may or may not be followed. Leader domination, or the equally troublesome loss of control, quickly undercuts enthusiasm and commitment.

5. *Cohesion.* Group members must be in harmony with the task and with concern for other members' values and positions. Divisive, prolonged conflict will undercut performance very quickly, not only in the group, but also at an organization-wide level. Attention must be given to the members. The care and nurturing of this social system is the means by which the group will accomplish its agenda. Formal structure and data are supporting players. Members' interactions are controlled. Leaders are expected to manage conflict, incorporate diverse opinions, and ensure that contributions are made from all members. No member is allowed to dominate, or pursue individual agendas at the expense of the group as a whole.

6. *Audience.* Is the consumer of the committee's work the administration, the medical staff, and/or outside stakeholders (e.g., accreditation teams or corporate purchasers)? Although there is much overlap, each audience has a different objective. Attention must be paid to the prime consumer first. A prepared and time-limited agenda must be distributed beforehand. Each leader must have a clear sense of what is to be accomplished at each meeting; this quite obvious need is frequently ignored because of the numerous competing demands for clinical time. Leaders must keep to the schedule by adhering to the predetermined meeting length while maintaining deadlines Long meetings and missed due dates signal that the group is drifting and likely to be ineffectual.

7. *Action.* The group takes action. Continual processing of documentation without forward movement, which is sometimes a weakness, quickly reduces member interest, and in this era of deepened competition, time is in short supply. This characteristic emphasizes that the purpose of the group is active quality improvement, not prolonged, paralyzing analysis. Many members complain that nothing comes out of their investment of time and energy on committees and teams. We can ask a simple question to test the action orientation of the group: "What will be started, stopped, maintained, increased, or decreased as a result of our group's work?" No action is certain to diminish both present and future participation.

8. *Follow-up.* The need here is to ask two questions: "What effect did our actions have?" and "What has been our year-long contribution to the organization's performance?" Attention to outcome is both reinforcing and informative. When visible impact is not apparent, the group must track back to diagnosis. Does the group look to see if its actions have the desired impact? This can be a simple test of the correctness of the diagnosis and plan. And it can be a lead-in to further work to be accomplished. Not all issues are addressed completely by the first action. A continuing cycle of diagnosis, planning, action, and evaluation is the model, and it is one that is consistent with our quality management philosophy and methods.

Many quality specialists are very experienced group leaders. Regardless of the level and standing of the leader, concern for group performance fundamentals is vital to group success—and we are not considering only employees and fellow clinicians. Involving patients is critical, particularly in recent years as the industry has moved to a patient-focused strategy, rather than one driven by providers and administrators.[47,48] Just exactly how do we use groups to involve patients in quality policymaking and in quality assessment and improvement activities? This is clearly not a new subject; consumer perspectives have been recognized.[49] We are already involving patients in the groups that focus on the management of medical quality. Here are some examples:

- Physicians increasingly share information and decisionmaking at the point of service, sometimes with groups of patients with the same disease.
- Systematic patient-satisfaction surveys are now widespread.
- Focus groups are used to create interactive discussion that targets service experiences.
- Patients have organized into advocacy and support groups.
- Patient ombudspersons and patient representatives take complaints and solve individual problems.
- Patients contribute to teams working on quality indicator selection and data use.
- Patients participate on problem-solving and quality improvement teams.

Notice that we are involving patients at different levels. On an individual level, patients can now assess their own experience with care. On a unit or departmental level, patients can contribute to quality improvement teams. And, on an institutional and system level, patients contribute to policymaking and future planning—most often in groups, underscoring again the quality leader's ability to build and manage diverse teams.

The quality of the group process is an important element in teams that have undertaken the task of medical quality management. As we examine the clinical work of medical teams in our quality improvement tasks, we can take some time for self-examination of the process of our quality management work. Members donate scarce resources—time, energy, and commitment—to this important work. They deserve groups that run efficiently and effectively—that is, at a high-quality level.

Strategy Formulation and Implementation

The health care quality leader must identify, analyze, and help to choose the lead strategies that will maintain and improve the institution's quality of medical and health care. This knowledge and skill can flow from the technology employed in the planning process, or can be much less formal. Strategy is the choosing of a *future direction*, the articulation of a *vision* or *destination* (i.e., a desired quality future) and the *decisions* needed to build success. In a changing health care environment, strategy is dynamic, not static. The quality leader is an advocate for medical quality during corporate strategy formulation and throughout strategy implementation. When we recognize that corporate strategic decisions affect medical quality, we understand why it is so important for the quality management leader to have a voice in the direction of the enterprise. We expect quality management leaders to be a part of the executive group and to understand how and why their contribution is helpful. This again underscores the movement from clinical quality assurance specialist to medical executive (i.e., partner in institutional leadership). We recognize that medical staff must push quality at the clinical service level and at the strategic level—the latter being the locus of large decisions affecting quality.

How many physicians would be surprised to hear that corporate strategy affects what they do with patients and colleagues? In the new century, physicians see little remaining separation between administrative decisionmaking and clinical services. Nevertheless, with this recognition, too few physicians are engaged in the ongoing strategic dialogue that determines the future of patient services, medical student teaching, and basic and applied research. Consider three fictitious but familiar examples of the impact of strategy on the quality of physicians' work:[50]

1. *Trauma center.* Hospital leaders were initially delighted to see the opening of their trauma center. Full accreditation made for good, "page one" coverage. After five years, however, the center's status was revisited. The cost of funding a trauma team with on-call surgeons and helicopter transport was very high. The number of trauma patients was dropping below the minimum required to maintain quality practices and skills. As the leadership team studied the center, they found that the clinical team was very competent but not outstanding. Two other trauma centers in the city were promoting their services aggressively. The executive team decided to eliminate the trauma center to concentrate on other clinical specialties. They believed that they were protecting the quality of the institution's services by focusing on what they did well.

2. *University hospital merger.* Two city hospitals merged as part of the greater development of United Health System. The university hospital held a national reputation for cutting-edge clinical research, outstanding teaching, and innovative service delivery. The United Health System now began to pressure faculty members to increase their clinical-revenue contribution. Faculty members became angry, as their "primary work" became clinical services. Teaching was now practically unfunded, and there were virtually no incentives to engage in research or educational activities. For the faculty members, the merger strategy clearly reduced the quality of their work.

3. *Solo to group.* Most, if not all, physicians recognize that the organization of medical practice is changing. Dr. David Donaldson practiced for 20 years by himself. As a small-town physician, he enjoyed his profession and was deeply attached to his community. As a nearby city grew to include his small town, he was invited to join a multispecialty group practice with 19 physician partners. He resisted at first, but the financial offer was attractive, and he was afraid of the changing environment. He made the change with many personal reservations, especially fearing the loss of physician-patient relationships. Six months later, he found that he now had collegial relations with his partners, better access to multidisciplinary services, informal consultation, a quality management system, and even a continuing-education series. On reflection, Dr. Donaldson felt that his strategic move to the group organization improved the quality of his professional life and his practice activities.

Strategy requires choosing a future direction and articulating a vision or destination and the decisions needed to build success: high-quality medical and health care practices and a desirable professional life. In a changing health care environment, strategy is dynamic, not static. These case summaries illustrate that medical quality is improved or undercut not just in examination and operating rooms but also in executive suites. Physicians aspiring to quality leadership are advocates for quality during strategy formulation and throughout strategy implementation. In each strategic and operational option, a changed future will most likely occur when an open participative process takes into consideration both clinical affairs and organizational architecture (see Figure 3–1). Once we recognize that strategic decisions affect quality, it becomes clear that quality management leaders must have a voice in the *direction* of the enterprise (strategy) and in the *execution* of the strategies (operations).

The double track concept requires quality leaders to attack problems and opportunities in two dimensions.[51,52] On *Track 1*—the whole organization level—leaders make a public and strategic commitment to improve quality (e.g., to improve medical and health care services throughout the organization). This "strategic level" of the procedure requires top leaders to promote the *strategic*

Figure 3–1   The Two Approaches to Health Care Organizational Improvement: Clinical and Total Quality Management Tracks

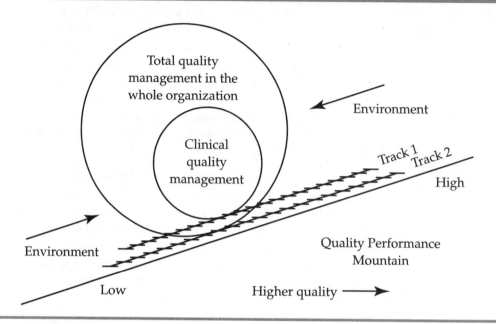

Clinical quality efforts (*Track 1*) are simulataneous with and part of total quality management (*Track 2*), which is helped and sometimes hindered by the external environment.

Source: From J. T. Ziegenfuss, *The Organizational Path to Health Care Quality.* Ann Arbor, Michigan: Health Administration Press/American College of Healthcare Executives Bks., 1993. Used with permission.

importance of redesign and create a vision of an improved quality future. This procedure is a well-established strategic planning and visioning path that has been used in the private sector for years. The emphasis here is on the choice of strategy and organizational architecture (e.g., incentives, authority, relations, and staffing).

Track 2 is the project (or team level) track, sometimes considered operations. This track involves very specific and operational problems (e.g., hospital discharge planning, operating-room turnover, how to inform poor families about immunization and nutrition needs, and placement procedures for recruiting and retaining rural physicians. Once a problem is identified, a team is formed and the questions quickly become: "What is our diagnosis of the problem?" and "What do we do?" Problem-solving procedures are followed as the team crafts specific solutions. There are numerous reports of re-engineering and quality improvement protocols to guide our efforts, some demonstrating breakthrough cases.[53] The traditional work of clinical quality assurance has been in this track, much of it developed in the past 15 years. We are now beginning to see research that explores the link between organizational culture and strategy (*Track 1*) and clinical outcomes (*Track 2*).[54]

The combined double track approach is based on several common purposes. Each of the procedures—quality improvement, re-engineering and visioning/strategic planning—is used for the following three purposes:

- evaluation and assessment (e.g., of current service delivery and of change impacts)
- teaching and learning (e.g., about health, the effectiveness and efficiency of service delivery models, and their processes)
- organization change and development (e.g., improvement in health care access)

This double track approach to strategy formulation and implementation is successful when quality leaders have portrayed their work as part of a learning community.[55] All members of the organization strive to continuously improve the quality of care by openly collecting and analyzing data about structures, processes, and outcomes regarding both strategic choice and operational success.

How can we further our understanding of our overall strategy—that is, the patterns of quality management work as a whole? What is it that we do in the medical organization to continue its growth and development? These questions intersect nicely with discussions in organization studies literature. In particular, the exploration of organizations as learning communities, or learning systems, has real potential to help us understand the contribution of quality specialists that becomes the endpoint of successful strategy formulation and implementation.

What is the connectedness? Quality improvement is at its base a learning process. We identify learning topics such as diseases, treatments, and delivery systems, and proceed to collect and analyze data to expand our knowledge of the subject. Beyond this basic commonality of purpose, there are additional connections that are best understood in the framework of the learning system concept. In 1995, Nevis, Dibella, and Gould listed what they believe are seven of the key elements that illustrate the orientation of the learning system, which is a combination of approach and practice.[56] We can see how quality management work in general fits these descriptors, and we can review this set in terms of our own individual efforts at our respective institutions.[57] To build learning communities, quality managers confront these seven design elements:

1. "*Knowledge source: internal–external:* Preference for developing knowledge internally versus preference for acquiring knowledge developed externally." Here, quality managers have an inclination to do both. Most would agree that internal data about medical quality is essential to an understanding of the uniqueness of that hospital or medical practice. But most also now agree that we can benefit from public and private benchmark data that allow us to put our own work in comparative context.

2. "*Product-process focus: What? How?:* Emphasis on accumulation of knowledge about what products/services are versus how organization develops, makes, and delivers its products/services." The debate over the importance of outcome versus process data has a long and rich history in quality management. We have come to recognize that we need both process and outcome information to both fully understand quality and move quality forward.

3. "*Documentation mode: personal–public:* Knowledge is something individuals possess versus publicly available know-how." The medical professions have long believed quality to be a personal and private issue. The "what and how" of medical practice has not been publicly available, but this situation is changing with increased demands from payers and from government funding of quality initiatives that offer public reports and analyses.

4. "*Dissemination mode: formal–informal:* Formal, prescribed, organization-wide methods of sharing learning versus informal methods such as role modeling and casual daily interaction." When we ask how quality feedback is given, in some practices the answer is "the same as always—informally and in private." Many medical organizations still retain this approach but they increasingly

have more formal means of presentation that are linked to credentialing, reappointment, and performance reviews.

5. *"Learning focus: incremental–transformative:* Incremental or corrective learning versus transformative or radical learning." Quality managers have learned to look for incremental gains and for strategic leaps. We can improve traditional cardiac bypass in small ways, radically re-engineer our approach to cardiac intervention with stents, or we can think of a transformation strategy such as the healthy community movement (i.e., moving from acute care to prevention).

6. *"Value-chain focus: design–deliver:* Emphasis on learning investments in engineering/production activities ("design and make" functions) versus sales/service activities ("market and deliver" functions)." Here, we find the quality management leaders now thinking about how to link present medical practice to the new developments of basic science and to the innovations found in both the academy and private practices. This interest lies on both the clinical and the delivery system sides, as it relates to how we diffuse innovation and encourage what we come to see as best practices.

7. *"Skill development focus: individual–group:* Development of individuals' skills versus team or group skills." Do we think of quality management as a solo or as a team endeavor? I think few would argue that quality improvement is a "lone wolf" practice. The complexities and disciplines involved ensure that teams are needed—teams that as a group become learning communities. Our medical and graduate schools increasingly recognize the importance of group skills and knowledge.

We have spent much of our quality management efforts on the core mission—planning for, controlling, and improving medical practices. While there has been some interest in reflecting on how this mission is accomplished, we could use more understanding of why and how quality management is effective. The work on learning systems may be a good opening for this exploration.

◉ Evaluation

The quality leader is constantly engaged in an effort to maintain and improve the quality of care provided. This evaluation effort is a critical aspect of the management role and is usually defined in terms of two purposes: *formative* and *summative*. Formative evaluation of medical care quality is designed to foster and support the ongoing improvement of quality of care, no matter what the level. Thus, nationally known departments already recognized for their high quality care ask what they need to do to become "world class." Local departments ask how they can become best in the region and in their particular marketplace. Data are developed to support, with facts, this continuous formative or developmental effort.

Leaders are also called on to help to make summative judgments about the quality of care, which is a performance-measurement mandate.[58] This evaluative work is not designed for development but for decisionmaking. If we decide that we have neither the resources nor the quality staff to provide a given type of care (e.g., trauma services), we can make a judgment based on benchmarks and internal clinical and financial data (e.g., volume, costs, and revenue) that trauma services should be dropped. Quality leaders are called on to help make tough decisions about what not to do based on indicators that drive performance.[59] The philosophy and methods of quality-of-care evaluation vary, depending on the evaluation purpose. Leaders must be able to engage in both formative and summative efforts that target all aspects of the organization. We expect quality leaders to offer "report cards" on their own quality efforts just as we look to see how our national efforts are faring.[60]

Leadership of quality management comprises the set of functions and roles that tie together the other elements of the organization's architecture. Managers are responsible for multisystem actions. In successful quality improvement programs, managers act to change all of the organization's elements, from structural incentives to clinical protocols to psychological climate and culture (sociotechnical impact). Readers should now be able to see the interrelatedness of the organizational systems architecture in the following statements about how quality management leaders build success in the quality improvement process:

- Increase employee and supervisor awareness of the need to change by continuously improving (psychosocial)
- Constantly reinforce the message that all processes can be improved (clinical-technical)
- Raise interest in quality by imposing an extensive period of orientation before implementation (psychosocial)
- Train a group of quality facilitators early, and assign them to teams (technical)
- Reinforce the idea that quality improvement applies to daily individual work as well as team efforts (technical)
- Celebrate quality successes (cultural)
- Have formal structures for chartering larger teams through a hospital-wide council (structure)
- Stay flexible (psychosocial; cultural)
- Create an atmosphere in which learning ways to improve a process is part of the job (cultural)

We can see that these points both summarize and reinforce the collective sense of a learning community—a community constantly searching for opportunities to improve.

Education Through Feedback

The development role of quality management leaders targets people *and* systems. For clinical and managerial personnel, development translates into an organization-wide staff-training program that is comprehensively implemented and highly competent. Crosby, Deming, and Juran all discuss the importance of investing in education. From the macro perspective (the whole unit or organization), support for organization-wide training requires an integrated view of individual and group development. Quite simply, if management does not develop people along with administration and clinical programs, the highly developed clinical and organizational processes will be run by underdeveloped personnel. Sooner or later, there will be a collapse in quality, or real quality improvement will be blocked by people lacking the necessary skills and knowledge.

Quality improvement occurs at the group level when the diagnosis-planning-action cycle is lean, simple, and can operate quickly. No elaborate forms or multiple sign-offs that can lead to long delays are present in the cycle. Although each of the quality improvement leaders—Deming, Juran, and Crosby—suggests careful data collection and analysis for which executives must be educated, each also has a bias against inaction that produces bureaucracy and delay.[61] With testing of underlying assumptions and the impact of actions taken, the learning can be a double loop moving beyond solving symptoms to addressing the root causes of deeper design problems.[62]

A final critical skill and knowledge base underlies this educational objective and many of the above activities. Quality leaders must know how to feed data and information back to their various constituencies, from administrative to clinical to corporate and regulatory audiences.[46] While this is a practical skill, it is of vital importance in situations where the data are sensitive and have strategic implications. Feedback techniques for survey and problem-solving data are not new topics; their use is vitally important during formative, developmental processes (i.e., the work of continuous quality improvement teams). Experienced quality leaders pay attention to and understand these aspects of the feedback transaction: purpose, clarity and specificity, descriptive—not evaluative—in nature, timeliness, participative interpretation, comparative basis for, situational security for audience, and action orientation. Each of these dimensions has been explored by practitioners and academics, particularly those in the field of organization change and development.

Harrison summarized the 10 critical characteristics of good feedback processes used in organizational change and development.[63] Adapted (with some substitutions) to fit the quality management task, the following nine points are worth our attention:

1. *Clarity of purpose.* Data can be used for development or for rendering judgment (formative versus summative, in evaluation research language). To use the data for continuing organizational development, the presenters and the audience must recognize that the purpose is a formative one. Learning and change to improve the care and delivery process is the goal. A judgmental purpose (summative) offers a figurative grade of pass or fail and if designed for this grading purpose will not serve the audience or the presenters.

2. *Clear and specific data.* Presented data must be relevant to the group or unit that receives it. For example, patient satisfaction data collected for the institution as a whole is rarely useful at the unit level unless enough patients are sampled to represent that particular unit. However, clinical teams are often asked to review satisfaction data in aggregate.

3. *Descriptive, not evaluative.* Useful feedback describes what is happening but does not offer an evaluative judgment (unless that is the intended purpose). The presenters must not rush into judgment without some interactive discussion with the audience.

4. *Timely.* How close to the action being reviewed are the data describing the events? The golden rule is quick feedback, which could mean monthly, quarterly, or semiyearly. Much quality data is older than one year, by which time behaviors and environment may have changed. Old data is useful for historical and longitudinal purposes but is not supportive of behavior change in the short term.

5. *Limited.* How great is the scope of the data? This characteristic requires that we tailor and focus the data to fit the specific, targeted needs of users. Data relevant to surgery quality do not include institutional financial trends, social work, or pharmacy department information. Although such information might be useful to hospital executives, surgeons need to focus on feedback regarding surgical outcomes and side effects.

6. *Comparative.* There is an ongoing debate about the usefulness of benchmarking and comparative data—they emphasize "followership," not leadership. But audiences want to know how they compare with others and with their own past performance. To leave out comparative information is to deprive the recipients of knowledge about their progress or lack thereof. This eliminates the ability to answer the question: "Are we improving?"

7. *Participative interpretation.* This condition reflects the notion that the final and complete analysis can be conducted without audience involvement. Joint interpretation is consistent with the developmental/formative purpose, as analysts and clinicians joined in the improvement task to discuss meaning and follow-up action.

8. *Safety and security.* Receiving performance feedback is both a technical and a psychological event. We need first to have the data correct (i.e., technical). It is important to recognize that all evaluations generate some anxiety. Presenters must be sensitive to the psychology of the process and offer language and behavior that protects the recipients.

9. *Practical and action oriented.* To be useful, the data should suggest some follow-up action and should be practical enough to be used by professionals in the field. Elite statistical analysis must be "walked across" to service-level implications. "What do the data tell us to do?" is the bottom-line question.

Most quality leaders have been providing evaluative feedback regarding the quality of health care delivery systems for some time. Many feel that they have learned the lessons noted in the previous nine points. But we may need to revisit our learning about the feedback process. Mistakes in presentation style, scope, clarity, and follow-up are common. Quality management leaders must recognize that the "art" of feedback is one of the critical skills of this work.

Organization and Management Summary

What do quality management leaders do? What do they value? And how does the quality management leader's role and behaviors fit into the complex organizations where many of us work? With a strong history in clinical quality assurance and interest in evidence-based medicine, we tend to take a technological view of quality management, focusing on data reliability and validity, samples, software, and other technical aspects regarding the assessment of quality. But quality is achieved by total organizational commitment, positive employee attitudes and psychological climate, involving patients, and targeting attention to quality objectives—the "softer side" of organization. Leaders are expected to know and be skilled in both dimensions, thus incorporating a *sociotechnical* perspective and skill set. We want leaders skilled at quantitative analysis as well as leaders capable of providing evidence of quality to regulators, litigants, and managed care negotiators. But those same leaders must know that the way in which quality is developed is through people. The core competencies comprise a blend of technical and interpersonal skills—a blend of expertise with diagnostic, teaching, and facilitative capability.

Quality management leaders use core competencies to fulfill key responsibilities for quality through various roles that have widespread organizational impact.

The quality effort in many organizations began as a response to complaints. Hospitals fostered the growth of quality programs, many of which have taken a whole-organization perspective through total quality management. Over the years, quality management has evolved in many health care organizations. Quality leaders now combine quality control with continuous problem-solving and change-agent activity. The day-to-day work of current quality specialists often involves three activities: (a) data analysis and problem-solving, (b) education and training, and (c) diagnostic and change consulting with senior management and clinicians. Clinicians and patients confront errors that are investigated and resolved inside the organization (i.e., without

Figure 3–2 Quality, Organizational Systems, and Leadership

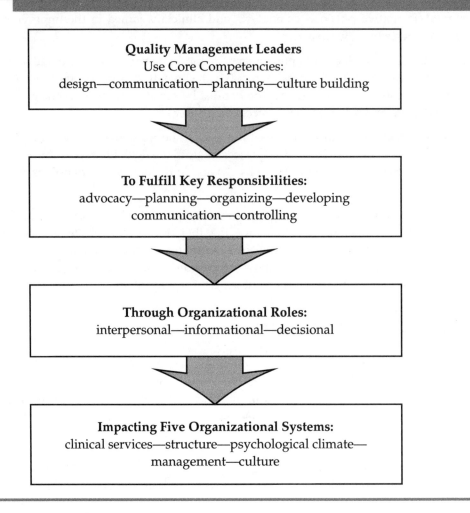

resorting to litigation). Quality management leaders use their knowledge of problem-solving and corporate policy and practice to contribute to prevention-oriented education and training. And, experienced quality leaders are able to inform senior management about opportunities for improvement as well as the problem patterns emerging, thus creating a "feedback loop" that identifies clinical and administrative policy and practice issues for attention.

What is the relationship of the work of quality leaders to organization design and to total quality thinking? We can return to our systems view; there are five links. Today, quality leaders:

1. *Expand the technical approach to quality.* Quality management in an organizational sense has increased the purview and impact of quality initiatives. Quality is enhanced by identifying and addressing organization-wide problems, with the analysis of the pattern of concerns leading to redesign and prevention (i.e., changed architecture). Quality management leaders see individual

cases, and the patterns of issues raised, as a source of information for developing both clinical services and the supporting organizational architecture.

2. *Create structural presence.* The permanent presence of quality management leaders demonstrates that the organizational structure includes elements that are representative of quality and problem-solving. When the quality management leader reports directly to the president/CEO, the authority-structure link is strong and clearly announces top management's concern for quality. This "structural addition" to the medical architecture ensures that there is someone able to cross departmental and hierarchical boundaries to address problems and pursue opportunities.

3. *Account for patient psychology.* Patients feel comforted when they receive care in organizations where quality is monitored and when they receive assistance in resolving conflicts. We have long known that medical malpractice litigation frequently begins when patients get angry about perceived versus real experiences. "Talk to me now or talk to me in court" is a reality. The uncertainty of critical illness is fertile ground for conflicts that add little value. Quality management leadership adds a human element to a system, dominated by high technology, where practitioners have scarce time to address problems in a civilized way. Quality is viewed as a social/psychological as well as a technical process.

4. *Support high-performance management.* The presence of quality management signifies that management is not afraid of data, including customer opinion and the challenge of continuous improvement. Several years ago, management experts suggested that we should "celebrate" the arrival of customer complaints, which translate, in quality language, as opportunities for improvement. We often recognize what we are doing well but receive too little negative feedback too late. In addition, senior executives are often sheltered from problems, for fear of "bringing death to the messenger." Analysis of quality indicators is part of the "database" needed to manage effectively—that is, continuously improve quality organization-wide. Managers factor in feedback as they create strategies and systems for the future.

5. *Reinforce and support culture values.* A quality management leader represents the company's values of equity, openness, internal responsiveness, and continuous improvement—all are characteristics of a high-performance company culture.[40] We intend that patients be treated fairly with regard to access to treatment, billing, benefit coverage, and communication. The "cultural heroes" of the modern health care company are those willing to openly respond to patient comments using the data to move forward, thus preventing future occurrences and redesigning patient care delivery systems. This systems thinking and leadership requires clinical staff to be knowledgeable about and skilled in organization design and administration.[64]

In summary, there are several key points supporting use of organizational thinking as part of the quality improvement effort. First, both the patient and clinical staff have a "voice" in an increasingly complex and competitive system. Second, quality management serves to promote equity and open problem-solving in quality-of-care and quality-of-life issues. Third, quality leaders provide data to move the organization forward. Finally, and most importantly, the presence of the quality management effort helps us to remember that no one creates a perfect organization. Although we continue to proactively strive for even better designs for delivering care, we have quality-of-care leaders able to help us address the social and technical flaws in existing systems while building the service architecture of the future.

References

1. Crosby PB. *Quality Is Free*. New York, NY: McGraw-Hill; 1979.

2. Deming WE. *Out of the Crisis*. Cambridge, MA: MIT, 1986.

3. Juran JM. *Juran on Leadership for Quality*. New York, NY: Free Press, 1989.

4. McLaughlin CP, Kaluzny AD. Total quality management in health: Making it work. *Health Care Management Review* 1990;15(3):7–14.

5. Ackoff RL. *A Concept of Corporate Planning*. New York, NY: Wiley; 1970.

6. Ackoff RL. *Creating the Corporate Future*. New York, NY: Wiley; 1981.

7. Berwick DM. Crossing the boundary: Changing mental models in the service of improvement. *International Journal for Quality in Health Care*. 1998;5(3):219–225.

8. Berwick, DM, Goffrey AB, Roessner J. *Curing Health Care*. San Francisco, CA: Jossey Bass, 1990.

9. Juran JM. Made in U.S.A.: A renaissance in quality. *Harv Bus Rev*. 1993;71(4):42–47,50.

10. Flood AB, Fennell ML. Through the lenses of organizational sociology: The role of organizational theory and research in conceptualizing and examining our health care system. *Journal of Health & Social Behavior*. 1995;Spec:154–169.

11. Pasmore WA. *Designing Effective Organizations: The Sociotechnical Systems Perspective*. New York, NY: Wiley; 1988.

12. Sirkin H, Stalk G, Jr. Fix the process, not the problem. *Harv. Bus. Rev*. 1990;68(4):26–33.

13. Kast FE, Rosenzweig, JE. *Organization and Management: A Systems and Contingency Approach*. New York, NY: McGraw-Hill, 1985. Fourth Edition.

14. Nadler DA, Gersteim MS, Shaw RB. *Organizational Architecture*. San Francisco, CA: Jossey Bass; 1992.

15. Ziegenfuss JT. *Organization and Management Problem Solving: A Systems and Consulting Approach*. Thousand Oaks, CA: Sage Books; 2002.

16. Goldfarb S. The utility of decision support, clinical guidelines, and financial incentives as tools to achieve improved clinical performance. *Joint Commission Journal on Quality Improvement*. 1999;25(3):137–144.

17. Kerr S. On the folly of rewarding A, while hoping for B; more on the folly. *Academy of Management Executive*. 1995;9(1)7–16.

18. Hammermeister KE. Participatory continuous improvement. *Annals of Thoracic Surgery*. 1994;58(6):1815–1821.

19. Mintzberg H. The manager's job: Folklore and fact. *Harv. Bus Rev*. 1975;49–61.

20. Senge PM. The leaders new work: Building learning organizations. *Sloan Management Rev*. Fall 1990;71–82.

21. Colenda CC, Wadland W, Hayes O, et al. Training tomorrow's clinicians today—managed care essentials: A process for curriculum development. *The American Journal of Managed Care*. 2000;6(5):561–572.

22. Blair JD, Payne GT. The paradox prescription: Leading the medical group of the future. *Health Care Management Review*. 2000;25(1):45–58.

23. Smircich L. Concepts of culture and organizational analysis. *Administrative Science Quarterly*. 1983;28,339–358.

24. Schein, EH. *Organizational Culture and Leadership*. San Francisco, CA: Jossey Bass, 1985.

25. Lundberg CC. Knowing and surfacing organizational culture: A consultant's guide. In: Golembiewski RT, ed. *Handbook of Organizational Consultation*. New York, NY: Marcel Dekker; 1993.

26. Ziegenfuss JT, Jr. Organizational barriers to quality improvement in medical and health care organizations. [Review] [41 refs]. *Quality Assurance & Utilization Review*. 1991;6(4):115–122.

27. Langlais RJ. Recognizing organizational impediments to the total quality management process. *Best Practices & Benchmarking in Healthcare*. 1996;1(1):16–20.

28. Reinertsen JL. Collaborating outside the box: When employers and providers take on environmental barriers to guideline implementation. *Joint Commission Journal on Quality Improvement*. 1995;21(11):612–618.

29. Reinhardt UE. The United States: Breakthroughs and waste. *Journal of Health Politics, Policy & Law*. 1992;17(4):637–666.

30. Dyer G. Am I using a systems approach? *Systems Practice*. 1993;6(4):407–419.

31. Ziegenfuss JT. Are you growing systems thinking managers? Use a systems model to teach and practice organizational analysis and planning, policy and development. *Systems Practice*. 1992;5(5):509–527.

32. Delbecq AL. Five leadership patterns for contemporary healthcare systems. *Emerging Issues in Healthcare*. Englewood, CO: Estes Park Institute; 1986.

33. Ziegenfuss JT. Five responsibilities of medical quality leaders. *Am J Med Qual*. 1997;12(4):175–176.

34. Ashkenas RN, Fracis SC. Integration managers: Special leaders for special times. *Hav Bus Rev*. 2000;78(6):108–116.

35. Bart CK, Tabone JC. Mission statements in Canadian not-for-profit hospitals: Does process matter? *Health Care Management Review*. 2000;25(2):74–84.

36. Ziegenfuss JT. Visioning, reengineering and continuous quality improvement: Parts of the quality management whole. *Am J Med Qual*. Winter 1998;13(4);173.

37. Walston SL, Rush MC. Altruistic organizational citizenship behavior: Context, disposition, and age. *Health Services Research*. 2000;34(6):1363–1388.

38. Luck J, Peabody JW. Improving the public sector: Can reengineering identify how to boost efficiency and effectiveness at a VA medical center? *Health Care Management Review*. 2000;25(2):34–44.

39. Hiatt A. Building corporate character [interview by Nan Stone]. *Harv Bus Rev*. 1992;70(2):94–104.

40. Collins JC, Porras JI. *Built to Last*. New York, NY: Harper Business, 1994.

41. Enthoven AC, Vorhaus CB. A vision of quality in health care deliver. *Health Affairs*. 1997;16(3):44–47.

42. Bates DW, Gawande AA. The impact of the Internet on quality measurement. *Health Affairs*. 2000;19(6): 104–114.

43. Conway AC, Keller RB, Wennberg DE. Partnering with physicians to achieve quality improvement. *Joint Commission Journal on Quality Improvement*. 1995;21(11):619–626.

44. Parcells B. The tough work of turning around a team. *Hav Bus Rev*. 2000;78(6):179–182.

45. Gardner DB, Cummings C. Total quality management and shared governance: Synergistic processes. *Nursing Administration Quarterly*. 1994;18(4):56–64.

46. Ziegenfuss JT. Quality management data: The feedback challenge. *Am J Med Qual*. 2000;15(2):47–48

47. Ford RC, Fottler MD. Creating customer-focused heath care organizations. *Health Care Management Review*. 2000;25(4):18–33.

48. McLaughlin CP, Kaluzny AD. Building client centered systems of care: Choosing a process direction for the next century. *Health Care Management Review*. 2000;25(1):73–82.

49. Cleary PD, Edgman-Levetan S. Health care quality. Incorporating consumer perspectives. *JAMA*. 1997; 278(19):1608–1612.

50. Ziegenfuss JT. The quality impact of business strategy. *Am J Med Qual*. September-October 1999;14(5)185.

51. Ziegenfuss JT. *The Organizational Path to Health Care Quality*. Ann Arbor, MI: Health Administration Press, 1993.

52. Ziegenfuss JT. Toward a general procedure for quality improvement. The double track process. *American Journal of Medical Quality*. 1994;9(2):90–97.

53. Nackel JG. Breakthrough delivery systems: Applying business process innovation. *Journal of the Society for Health Systems*. 1995;5(1):11–21.

54. Shortell SM, Jones RH, Rademaker AW, et al. Assessing the impact of total quality management and organizational culture on multiple outcomes of care for coronary artery bypass graft surgery patients. *Medical Care*. 2000;38(2):207–217.

55. Garvin DA. Building a learning organization. *Harv Bus Rev*. 1993;71(4):78–91.

56. Nevis EC, Dibella AJ. Gould JM. Understanding organizations as learning systems. *Sloan Management Review*. Winter 1995; 73–85.

57. Ziegenfuss JT. Quality management as a learning system. *Am J Med Qual*. 2001;169(3);79–80.

58. Eccles RG. The performance measurement manifesto. *Harv Bus Rev*. 1991;69(1):131–137.

59. Kaplan RS, Norton DP. The balanced scorecard—measures that drive performance. *Harv Bus Rev*. 1992;70(1):71–79.

60. Blumenthal D, Kilo CM. A report card on continuous quality improvement. [Review] [29 refs]. *Milbank Quarterly*. 1998;76(4):511, 625–648.

61. Skibicki R. Education executives to integrate information management with quality improvement: A case study. *Joint Commission Journal on Quality Improvement*. 1994;20(11):623–630.

62. Elliott RL. Double loop learning and the quality of quality improvement. *Joint Commission Journal on Quality Improvement*. 1996;22(1):59–66.

63. Harrison MI. *Diagnosing Organizations: Methods, Models and Processes*. 2nd ed. Thousand Oaks, CA: Sage; 1994; p76.

64. Ziegenfuss JT, Sassani J. (Eds.). *Portable Health Administration*. London, England: Academic Press, Elsevier Books; 2004.

● Related Readings

Anctil B, Winters M. Linking customer judgments with process measures to improve access to ambulatory care. *Joint Commission Journal on Quality Improvement*. 1996; 22(5):345–357.

Begun, JW, Luke RD. Factors underlying organizational change in local health care markets, 1982–1995. *Health Care Management Review*. 2001;26(2):62–72.

Blumenthal D, Edward N. A tale of two systems: The changing academic health center. *Health Affairs*. 2000;19(3):86–101.

Bossidy L. The job no CEO should delegate. *Hav Bus Rev*. 2001;79(3):46–49, 163.

Checkland P. *Systems Thinking, Systems Practice*. New York, NY: Wiley; 1981.

Chisholm R, Ziengefuss JT. Applying the sociotechnical systems approach to health care organizations. *Journal of Applied Behavior Science*. 1986;22(3):315–327.

Goldsmith J. The Internet and managed care: A new wave of innovation. *Health Affairs*. 2000;19(6):42–56.

Hofer TP, Hayward RA, Greenfield S, Wagner EH, Kaplan SH, Manning WG. The unreliability of individual physician "report cards" for assessing the costs and quality of care of a chronic disease. *JAMA*. 1999;281(22):2098–2105.

Kazandjian VA, Thomson RG, Law WR, Waldron K. Do performance indicators make a difference? *Joint Commission Journal on Quality Improvement*. 1996;22(7):482–491.

Keating CB. A systems-based methodology for structural analysis of health care operations." *Journal of Management in Medicine*. 2000;14(3–4):170–198.

Kritchevsky SB, Simmons BP. Continuous quality improvement. Concepts and applications for physician care. *JAMA*. 1991;266(13):1817–1823.

Landon BE, Wilson IB, Cleary PD. A conceptual model of the effects of health care organizations on the quality of medical care. *JAMA*. 1998;279(17):1377–1382.

Lesser CS, Ginsburg PB. Update on the nation's health care system: 1997–1999. *Health Affairs*. 2000;19(6)206–216.

Maxwell C, Ziegenfuss JT, Chisholm RF. Beyond quality improvement teams: Sociotechnical systems theory and self-directed work teams. *Quality Management in Health Care*. 1993;1(2):59–67.

McLaughlin CP. Balancing collaboration and competition: The Kingsport, Tennessee experience. *Joint Commission Journal on Quality Improvement*. 1995;21(11):646–655.

Nackel JG. Breakthrough delivery systems: Applying business process innovation. *Journal of the Society for Health Systems*. 1995;5(1):11–21.

Prahalad CK, Krishnam MS. The new meaning of quality in the information age. *Harv Bus Rev*. 1999;77(5): 109–118, 184.

Schein EH. Culture: The missing concept in organizational studies. *Administrative Science Quarterly*, 1996;11(2): 229–240.

Schein EH. Three cultures of management: The key to organization. *Sloan Management Review*, 1996;38(1):9–20.

Schein EH. *Organizational Culture and Leadership*. 2nd ed., San Francisco, CA: Jossey-Bass Publishers.

Shortell SM, Bazzoli GJ, Dubbs NL, Kralovec P. Classifying health networks and systems: Managerial and policy implications. *Health Care Management Review*. 2000;25(4):9–17.

Weil TP. Management of integrated delivery systems in the next decade. *Health Care Management Review*. 2000;25(3):9–23.

Wyszewianski L. Quality of care: Past achievements and future challenges. *Inquiry*. Spring 1988;25(1):13–24.

Chapter 4

ECONOMICS, FINANCE, AND GOVERNMENT IN MEDICAL QUALITY MANAGEMENT

Donald Fetterolf, MD, MBA

Joseph L. Braun, MD, JD, MBA

● Introduction

Throughout the past 10 years, economic, financial, and governmental issues have had an increasingly important influence on medical quality programs in the United States. Twenty years ago, medical quality efforts focused primarily on improving medical care delivery and enhancing clinical performance locally. As emerging models of *continuous quality improvement* transformed the business world, some of those concepts began, in turn, to affect the medical quality community.[1–7] Clinicians began to turn their attention from quality *assessment* (in which the quality of medical care was monitored primarily by case review) to continuous quality *improvement* (in which statistical quality control was used to monitor processes and improve outcomes).

For the purposes of this text, we might ask, "What is the general relationship between medical quality initiatives and the business world? How can activities in these two major realms influence each other? What critical insights or pieces of information do medical quality managers need in our current environment?"

Quality professionals are increasingly asked to "bring their expertise to the table" when solving important economic health care issues of the early 21st century and, specifically, when addressing concerns about rapidly rising health care costs. It is widely held that "higher quality costs less," and quality improvement efforts have been proposed as one method for reducing skyrocketing health care costs. As quality managers are asked to select medical management activities that are cost-effective, it is becoming apparent that higher quality sometimes costs *more* (although perhaps less than the same thing done poorly). As the next generation of quality management proceeds, medical quality managers are facing a trade-off between some elements of quality and the costs that can be absorbed by a society that continuously seeks to improve the health of its populations.[8–11] Indeed, newer approaches for reviewing the value of quality initiatives are multidisciplinary and consider financial, clinical, operational, as well as a variety of intangible variables. Quality professionals are also asked on a daily basis to evaluate issues involving errors in medicine, decreased patient satisfaction, and the evaluation of emerging technologies, and to make a variety of other critical decisions related to the adequacy and appropriateness of care.[12–14] In addition, quality professionals are continually being asked to identify new techniques and methods to improve the care delivery infrastructure. These issues are all inextricably entwined in the economic fabric of our society. The greatest current challenge is to balance a business-oriented focus on short-term financial outcomes with a medically oriented focus on the long-term gains created by quality improvement methods. Finally, increasing pressure to document the return on investment of quality improvement activities is being applied by the payer community. Large-company benefit managers typically demand to know what the return on investment is for clinical quality improvement activities and whether or not these activities are worth purchasing as part of the medical benefits for their employees.[15]

One definition of the mission of medical quality is to provide "quicker, cheaper, and better services." However, the resources available to a society—to provide health care to its citizens—are limited. Physicians who are responsible for quality management and involved in the economics, finance, and politics of health care must understand that a major planned—or even unexpected—change in any one of these fields will probably affect the other two. Predicting the result of these dynamics becomes astronomically more complicated when the outcome is not definitive or even tangible, but rather is a consequence of shifting resources that affect the cost of health care, alter the quality of health care, or impinge on access to health care. Even then, the dynamics can be viewed from, or measured at, multiple levels that are not necessarily consistent or even comparable.

The perspective of individuals involved in the overall health care process is also an important variable. The preferred health care outcome for an individual may not be the one desired by the director of the state Medicaid program, or the one promised by the administrator of the Center for Medicare Services at the Senate confirmation hearings. Patient-based, shared decisionmaking is emerging as another important variable, as the perspective of health care consumers must now be considered as well. Wide variation in the use of services begs the question as to the "correct" rate that should be applied. Absent evidence-based direction for all available therapies suggests that, for now, the "ideal" rate will be defined as the rate that will occur when individuals are each provided with all of the available information they need. As the complexity of clinical decisionmaking rises at both the individual and societal levels, medical quality practitioners must be familiar with concepts in economics, accounting, and government, as various evolving strategies deal with the combined crises of quality and affordability. Practitioners will often be called on to use quantitative methods to analyze processes and justify changes in terms of monetary factors, political expediency, and improved efficiency.

Several key questions introduce the substance of this chapter:

1. What is the relationship among policy, ethics, politics, law, and government?
2. What are the general business principles and key concepts in economic theory that the medical quality practitioner needs to understand?
3. What are some of the key financial and accounting concepts with which a medical quality practitioner must become familiar? How are these tools being used in new models of care-delivery analysis and operations?

4. What economic and policy events caused the government to become involved with medical care, and particularly, with medical quality?

5. What role do American values and health policy play, with regard to how medical quality practitioners should approach their tasks?

6. What is meant by "public good," and how does this concept apply to the role of the medical quality practitioner and the manner in which American society and government approach health care?

In this chapter, we address the above questions by reviewing the fundamentals of the economics, finance, and politics of medical quality in national, state, and local terms, and then illustrating how these three fields interact.

Historical Perspective

As noted above, the evolution of medical quality efforts in the United States has in many ways paralleled similar developments in the business world. Quality-oriented activities have progressed from an inspection-based approach to more modern, data-driven, analytic methods and principles of statistical quality control. At the same time, the approach of medical quality professionals has become increasingly entwined in a variety of business activities. The evolution of this process can be divided into four fairly distinct stages: (1) quality assurance, (2) statistical quality control and the notion of continuous quality improvement, (3) outcomes-focused analysis, and, finally, (4) fluid change.

1. *Stage 1: Quality assurance.* Efforts to improve quality in health care institutions followed an "inspection" mode for many years during the first part of the 20th century. Weekly "clinical pathology conferences," in which individual cases were presented and then reviewed at length, were common in hospitals and medical schools. During this time, medical departments typically concentrated on individual chart reviews, focusing on outlier cases for evaluation, and increased scrutiny. Inspection technologies were also common in the manufacturing arena during this period, before Shewhart and Deming introduced a number of statistical quality control techniques.[7, 16] Clinical activities focused on monitoring sentinel events, reviewing individual case studies, obtaining external accreditation, and looking for adverse outcomes in less systematic ways. In addition, Donabedian and others began to develop quality paradigms that focused on outcomes in medicine that would pave the way for the next stage in the development of the art.[4]

2. *Stage 2: Statistical quality control and the notion of continuous quality improvement.* In the next stage in the development of medical quality programs, efforts followed manufacturing and industry approaches for adopting statistical quality methods, such as control charts, to improve performance to specification. This period in medicine, which began in the 1980s, moved the focus from individual inspection to more systemic, statistical views of medical processes. The medical management community quickly adopted many of the statistical quality control or continuous quality improvement (CQI) techniques being developed by Deming and Shewhart.[7, 16] It was widely held in both industry and health care that many key distributions were "normal" (or "bell-shaped") distributions and that focusing on outlier activities could reduce variation and improve overall quality. Arguments that each patient was unique gave way to the view that health care could be analyzed in a systematic fashion. Analyses now included even more complex, multivariate or mul-

tidimensional analyses, made possible by increasing computing power and training of clinical analysts.

Excellent work was performed during this period to document statistical variation in health care delivery and clinical practice and to educate the medical community.[3, 9, 17, 18] Physicians' actions came to be seen as part of processes that could be modified through root-cause process change rather than through individual punitive measures. Analysis of variation in surgical procedure rates and results, as well as the development of preventive service standards, variation-based claims analyses, and clinical pathways or guidelines, were elevated to public view during this period. Providing feedback to physicians about these statistics was seen as the solution to many quality-related issues.

3. *Stage 3: Outcomes-focused analysis.* During the third stage in the evolution of quality management, the focus moved quickly to true outcomes. Not only were processes noted to have "bell curve" distributions, but it was believed that the mean, or center, portion of the bell curve could also be moved to higher levels of quality by manipulating the system on the high and low ends of the curve. Removing unnecessary variation in health care was seen as the solution to quality problems in this era, as measurement and reporting were linked to outcomes measures derived from evidence-based guidelines. As processes improved, less variation could be documented across processes, and "low outliers" on quality analyses were reduced.

Analyses also extended beyond simple engineering views of process. Objects of analysis focused on interventions that would change the course of illness, rather than on statistics such as admission rates. Measures included the application of preventive medicine and broader outcomes-based measures. Here, functional status evaluation, patients' perceptions of illness, and focus on disability and absenteeism emerged as important quality deliverables. Costs in health care were seen as decreasing, not only because variation was being reduced, but also because the very fabric of health care for individuals was being changed at the same time.

Higher-order thinking about the delivery system itself was adopted as a result of these more complex applications of quality measures. This period saw the development of hospital-physician joint ventures (PHOs), physician networks, community health information networks (CHINs), and "integrated delivery systems" (IDSs). It was believed that widespread integration and coordination of activities could not only reduce variation but also improve care through improved communication and process refinement.[19] Unfortunately, for a variety of reasons, the large savings in health care costs, and improvements in quality, were not universally realized, and many of these structures were disassembled.

Also during this period, intensive oversight developed to ensure that the new tools were applied. The Joint Commission on the Accreditation of Healthcare Organizations (JCAHO), the American Accreditation Healthcare Commission (URAC), and the National Committee for Quality Assurance (NCQA) became large dominant organizations in the oversight of quality processes. Large process-heavy bureaucracies, developed to support the demands of these organizations, were in turn increasingly recognized as quasi-governmental systems in the ongoing drive to assure quality. These organizations were supplemented and complemented by an expanding number of legislative and regulatory requirements that transformed the pursuit of medical quality into a compliance-focused mandate for many organizations. The Centers for Medicare and Medicaid Services (CMS) and the Food and Drug Administration (FDA) also increased their influence on the development of medical quality initiatives and the reimbursement of medical services.[20]

During the 1990s, the number of organizations that claimed importance in assuring quality activities rapidly expanded (see Table 4–1). Hospitals, health plans, governmental agencies, and physicians found themselves increasingly entangled in this large medical bureaucracy that sought to assure quality by using a variety of earlier tools.

4. *Current Stage (Stage 4): Fluid change.* Currently, another movement appears to be occurring in the evolution of quality improvement activities, as society begins to focus simultaneously on the burden created by quality improvement accreditation and on the loss of control over rising medical costs. Current efforts are designed to maximize clinical effects by adopting evidence-based

Table 4–1	Examples of External Organizations Concerned About Health Care Quality

Governmental

Agency for Healthcare Research and Quality (AHRQ)
Centers for Medicare and Medicaid Services (CMS)
Peer review organizations ("PROs")
Quality improvement organizations ("QIOs")
State departments of health
State departments of insurance

Accreditation

Accreditation Association for Ambulatory Health Care (AAAHC)
American Accreditation Healthcare Commission (URAC)
Joint Commission for the Accreditation of Healthcare Organizations (JCAHO) and the ORYX measures
National Committee for Quality Assurance (NCQA); includes use of Health Plan Employer Data and Information Set (HEDIS) and Consumer Assessment for Health Plans Study (CAHPS) tools

Business

Business Health Care and Purchasing Coalitions
    (1) Washington Business Group on Health
    (2) Pacific Business Group on Health
Foundation for Accountability (FAcct)
Leapfrog Group
Local business groups and councils
National Business Coalition on Health

Others

American Association of Health Plans (AAHP)
Blue Cross/Blue Shield Association (BCBSA)
Council for Affordable Quality Healthcare (CAQH)
Doctors Office Quality Project (DOQ)
Institute of Medicine (IOM)
National Quality Forum (NQF)
Organized medical associations (e.g., American Medical Association)
Professional organizations (e.g., American Heart Association)
Specialty societies (sources of guidelines and recommendations; e.g., the American College of Cardiology, working with the American Heart Association)

guidelines, and organizations are being created to develop and test these guidelines, and to certify practitioners in many disciplines.

Evidence-based consensus conferences have increasingly dictated which areas of focus that organizations should follow, and how care should be delivered. Although this approach represents an improved direction for care delivery, the sheer number of guidelines makes it impossible for an individual practitioner to stay current.

Recently, accreditation bodies have presented large volumes of "standards" that must be perused and followed. There is widespread frustration as well as a belief in the payer community that all of this costly activity may not be rapidly addressing fundamental issues, such as reducing errors in medicine or containing the rising cost of health care. At the same time, government interest in improving quality has led to the government's imprimatur of accreditation agencies and the simultaneous loading of the system with additional quality requirements generated by government agencies. As we move into the first decade of the 21st century, it is likely that the plethora of standards, guidelines, and demands will need to be consolidated. A number of organizations, such as the National Quality Forum, are working to achieve this goal.

Physician-level public reporting of clinical outcomes has been discussed for a number of years, but with increasing shifts to consumer-driven health care programs and better availability of data, the public is questioning why more information is not made accessible. Subtle, important nuances in interpreting health care data—that are well known to statisticians and physicians—are viewed as roadblocks by the public in their quest to find good physicians and to eliminate ineffective or dangerous practitioners. Public pressure will certainly accelerate public disclosure, but with uncertain results.

Simultaneously, consolidating large data sets in enterprise data warehouses in government and insurer organizations has led to the possibility that informatics-driven evaluation of process may build on previous activities as well. Predictive modeling, data mining, and the application of a variety of sophisticated techniques for locating and abstracting information related to medical quality initiatives are occurring at unprecedented rates (see Box 4–1).

| Box 4–1 | Discussion: Health plan use of predictive modeling in quality improvement activities |

Health plans have recently compiled large databases of claims in "enterprise data warehouses." In what was once a one-claim-at-a-time transaction-processing environment, sophisticated analysts are now being hired to "mine" the data. In one type of data-mining technique, analysts aggregate plan members into similar "clusters" using complicated statistical algorithms generated in complex analytic software programs. Individual clusters are designed to be clinically relevant and to allow targeted medical quality interventions. A program of this type might identify people with diabetes who have a history of consulting a renal specialist and undergoing kidney function testing at a certain frequency, indicating that they are members of a group likely to have high future medical costs. Clinical interventions designed to improve quality by diagnosing, at an early stage, impending renal failure in patients with diabetes, or by improving the medication compliance of patients with asthma, are direct consequences of these types of sophisticated tools.

Looking to the future, quality professionals in the early 21st century must have not only a basic understanding of the definitions of quality under various scenarios and how quality can be improved using various tools, but also a deep knowledge of how the quality industry and the "medical quality bureaucracy" are leading the economy and the efforts of quality professionals. Skills needed by quality professionals include an understanding of compliance, informatics, health services research, regulatory history, and organizational psychology. In the United States, we have moved from small, community-based efforts to large, integrated national initiatives that seek to alter substantially the quality of care in numerous defined ways. Quality professionals must integrate governmental control and mandates, economic changes in the health care delivery infrastructure, political pressures, and constrained resources in an ever-challenging manner.

Basic Concepts in Business and Economics

Delivering an in-depth knowledge of business economics and finance is beyond the purview of a single chapter in a book directed at entry-level training for quality professionals. Yet this knowledge has become increasingly important for all health care professionals. Physicians and nurses in record numbers are pursuing master's degrees in business, public management, and similar disciplines to cope with the increasing integration of economic concerns in the health care industry. The main categories of economics, accounting, and finance are worth reviewing briefly, particularly as they relate to quality professionals.

Economics

Uninformed students are often deterred from studying economics by its reputation for being difficult and complicated. In fact, economics offers a fascinating insight into the way that the social world around us moves and operates.

Business schools divide the study of economics into *macroeconomics* and *microeconomics*. Macroeconomics typically deals with the "big picture" of the structure and performance of the industrial market and the behavior of society at large. The money supply, and how it affects wages, prices, employment, inflation, and long-term growth and productivity, comprise a major part of this topic. Macroeconomics is mainly focused on the behavior of the economy as a whole and its total output and activity at the national or international level. It also deals with these activities over time and how they affect the wealth of nations and overall business cycles.

Macroeconomics usually focuses on the markets in general, rather than on a specific region or product, but it can still be applied locally. Students of the subject recognize that it is an inexact science that has developed a variety of different approaches. Keynesian economics was developed in the earlier part of the 20th century, and its tenets were frequently considered guiding principles until the late 20th century. The Keynesian approach has since been supplemented by a variety of theoretical constructs that continue to evolve.

Regulation of the monetary supply through the Federal Reserve Board presents a "monetarist" approach to economics that is relatively recent and that has been fueled by complex econometric computer models. Considerable disagreement arises among various schools of economics as to what the best approach may be, how the market responds to various drivers, and what a government's best course of action may be. These theories are also influenced in part by the political views of individual analysts who might emphasize, for example, the role of business and organizations over the perceived need to improve the quality of life for the general public.

Economics develops methods of understanding the best ways to do things, given certain observations, but it often delivers several options. Economists might say, for example, that rent controls cause perturbations in the market that are unintended and that the approach is suboptimal. They might suggest that a more rational and direct approach to improving housing disparities would yield other possibilities, such as providing rent vouchers, creating zoning rules mandating that a portion of all housing in an area contain small apartments, or raising wages through education. The choice of approach would still depend on political views, but the science of economics proposes that more efficient approaches be favored over those with more problematic consequences.

A common misunderstanding among clinically trained health care professionals is that economics is all about money. In fact, economics focuses on the creation, evolution, and delivery of *value*, which may include (1) non-monetary elements, such as labor forces, (2) factors that alter the business cycle, (3) the influence of history, and (4) the general thoughts and motives of the population in the aggregate.

A more than passing understanding of economics is useful for health care professionals, particularly as the continual rise in health care costs increasingly influences the economy. The health care system as a whole is clearly an issue in macroeconomics, now that the overall cost of health care is 15% of the gross national product of the United States. As the health care delivery system has expanded, it has assumed an increasingly large role in the economy overall, including manufacturing, labor, and the economies of governments.

Economists have noted a close relationship between consumption spending and disposable income.[21] Current trends in the use of disposable income in health care spending are unsustainable from a mathematical perspective. Historical changes in the US economy during economic recessions have also resulted in considerable pressure on large businesses to reduce health care expenditures as they become an increasing portion of a company's expenses, thus making the company less competitive in world markets. An understanding of the structure of macroeconomics is useful for quality professionals because the economic environment in health care becomes increasingly complicated.

The second portion of the course work in economics focuses on microeconomics, or "the economics of the firm." In contrast to macroeconomics, which centers on industrial market structure and performance, microeconomics becomes interested in the effects of these various forces on individual firms and regions or market segments. In health care, microeconomic studies focus on individual physician practices, the workings of hospital markets and service areas, and the nuances of physician payment systems. Market demand and demand curves are of interest to individual companies seeking to set the price and volume of services they offer. This area of economics is clearly relevant to a medical care system that has been growing during the past five decades, particularly with the support of government subsidies.

Microeconomics is also concerned with the behavior of individuals as they relate to an organization. How individuals view the price of a company's service is related to the utility that they attribute to these services. In organizations that appear to be offering commodities—and health care is increasingly being positioned as a commodity—payers at the individual or business level may be indifferent about which provider is used and will move to higher prices or different providers only through more complex relationships that alter demand.

Microeconomic analysis can evaluate consumer behavior regarding the purchase of health care services. Large insurance carriers do market research, then mathematically review ways in which consumer behavior can be altered, such as through various types of charges and perceived quality. Insurers and payers are interested, for example, in the types of incentives that may change the like-

Box 4–2	Discussion: Price elasticity of demand among purchasers of health insurance services

Insurers—indeed sellers of many products—note that certain price points will move customers in the direction of their product. For example, insurers and managed care organizations report that as little as $10-per-member-per-month out-of-pocket cost can cause a consumer to shift from one type of health provider to another. Physicians are often firmly convinced that their patients will come to them forever, because they believe that the definitive bond is the relationship between the doctor and the patient. Actual practice, however, suggests that to obtain a savings of $8 to $10 per member per month, a consumer will shift to a different physician. The more easily the patient can shift plans and networks, the more "elastic" is the relationship between individuals and the choice of purchasing services by a given physician. Many factors affect the elasticity of demand, such as: (1) the presence of equivalent substitutes (the perception among some patients that all doctors are equal or offer commodity services); (2) penetration of the product into the community (patients will pick HMOs if many are available in the marketplace, but may be less inclined to do so when managed care develops in an indemnity market), or perceived differences in quality; (3) income profile of the consumer purchasing the product, etc.

lihood that consumers will seek health services, particularly as this likelihood relates to pricing—the so-called *price elasticity of demand* (see Box 4–2).

The response of individuals in *monopoly* or *monopsony* markets is also of interest to large insurance carriers, in both *highly concentrated* and *unconcentrated* labor markets. In a monopoly, a seller represents a dominant or unique vendor of services. Prices for services can be set higher than in more competitive markets. In highly concentrated markets, which have only a few insurers for a region, individuals and businesses may complain that this effect is what is making their premiums high. They may state that high "barriers to entry" in the market prevent the health care competition from decreasing prices. Similar complaints arise when a "sole community provider" of health care services, such as a regional rural hospital, negotiates higher fees for its services with a health plan.

In a monopsony, the purchaser of services represents a unique or dominant position in the market (see Box 4–3). The federal government with respect to Medicare services can be thought of as a monopsony, as might a dominant employer in a region. The effects in this case also concern the public and government officials as the costs of health care rise. This issue is of concern to physicians, who represent a segment of the labor force that must contract with various organizations. For example, the behavior of primary care and specialist physicians is likely to vary in different types of markets, depending on the level of the physicians' market control. In markets with a dominant insurer and an oversupply or undersupply of a particular type of physician specialty, these factors greatly affect the physicians' interpretation of how aggressive they can be with the payer. Physicians in short supply and in high demand can negotiate higher-than-normal fees for their services. Physicians in more plentiful supply might in turn feel more downward pressure on their fees; they become *price takers*. In markets that are highly fragmented across many payers, the behavior of physicians and insurers would again vary according to whether physician specialties are over- or underrepresented.

> ### Box 4–3   Example: "Any willing provider" legislation: a direct consequence of insurers exerting monopsony powers
>
> Beginning in the 1990s, large consolidated payers of provider services in the United States determined that they would contract only with physicians and pharmacists who met certain price points. Large organized corporations were able to deliver these services through group purchasing, salary contracts, and a variety of other mechanisms, at prices that hurt individual practitioners or stores. In a successful lobbying effort, pharmacy stores argued that such actions essentially were hostile to the development of competition and free markets. In the mid 1990s, "any willing provider" legislation was proposed and passed regionally, allowing providers of services to continue to participate with the payers if they met a reasonable set of market requirements.

At about the same time, a similar situation arose in areas with an oversupply of certain types of health care providers (e.g., ophthalmologists or chiropractors). Because of their considerable market power, payers were able to specify the number of providers that they would allow into their health plans, stating, for example, that they "needed only 72 specialists" of a certain type in a region that had 150 or 200 such practitioners. The remaining practitioners were essentially disenfranchised from the payers' networks and were forced to face a smaller patient base. In markets in which insurers developed such a heavy market penetration, these economic forces drove specialists to engage in political activity that led to the passage of "any willing provider" legislation, which mandated that any provider who met basic criteria could be admitted to a network roster. Thus, the insurers' initial efforts to constrain overuse of certain services were met by market forces that resulted in increased access to providers of these services.

Clearly, the leverage that a payer or health plan has over physicians is also related to economic forces. How closely physicians are tied to a health plan directly influences their need or desire to participate in mandated quality initiatives. The economics of the behaviors of patients and providers has been studied with much interest. Textbooks that combine micro- and macroeconomics and a solid knowledge of the health care system are worth reviewing by medical care professionals of all types—and by quality professionals in particular.[10, 11, 22–25]

In conclusion, the importance of economics to health care professionals in general, and to quality managers in particular, is becoming increasingly evident as the overall effect of the health care system on the general economy becomes more prominent and more acute. Understanding economic forces and their relationship to the business community is an important capability needed at all levels of management in health care organizations. Training in economics can be obtained through graduate-level courses, although several less difficult avenues are available, such as intensive short courses offered by graduate business schools, brief introductory training sessions offered through professional societies, and audio learning tapes.[26] Health economics has developed into a specialty in its own right, and entire texts are available on the subject.[22,27,28]

Accounting

Why do quality management professionals need to develop a working knowledge of accounting, let alone take a course in this subject? The answer is that basic accounting principles are used in a variety of analyses and comprise the "language of business." Accounting is the main method used to record and present business transactions to other business professionals in order to communicate cost and movement of money. Although health professionals do not need to perform accounting procedures, they still must understand and appreciate basic accounting principles in much the same way that those pursuing internal medicine rather than surgery must have a thorough knowledge of anatomy.

Types of Financial Reporting Tools.

Medical quality managers are called on to review and understand the significance of a wide variety of financial information. Financial information can take many forms in a health plan or hospital (see Table 4–2). The main classes of financial, or accounting, reports are balance sheets, income statements, and statements of cash flow. Annual reports may contain any or all of these items.

1. *Financial statements.* Financial statements include the balance sheet, income statement, statement of cash flows, and similar documents. Courses in *financial accounting*, typically taught in business schools, provide instruction in how to prepare these statements, which are used to communicate with external publics, such as the Internal Revenue Service, auditors, and state governments.

Important features of financial statements are often expressed as ratios. These ratios include the *current ratio* (current assets divided by current liabilities), the *quick ratio* (current assets minus inventories over current liabilities), and various forms of debt and profit ratios. These statistics provide an estimate of how "solid" the company is, or whether its assets are sufficient to cover the debt it carries. Similar ratios reflect the return on activity of the company; for example, *return on investment* (ROI), *return on assets* (ROA), *return on equity* (ROE), and *earnings per share* (EPS) of stock are typically used. In these statistics, the amount of net earnings, or revenue, is divided by the numbers used for summarizing the asset base, outstanding equity, or by outstanding shares of stock, respectively. For medical managers, the most frequently requested statistic is the *return on investment*—the amount of

Table 4–2 Typical Forms of Financial Information

Financial statements
Annual reports
Budgets
Invoices
Bank statements
Sales forecast results
Financial forecast results
Claims payment records
Billed and paid premium records
General ledgers
Investment reports
Financial models
Cost accounting reports
Actual versus budget results for provider risk pools
Medical loss ratio and expense ratio reports
Utilization statistics reports
Payroll records

Source: Academy for Healthcare Management. Health Plan Finance and Risk Management. Atlanta, GA. Academy for Healthcare Management. 1999.[46]

money returning to the organization for the financial investment in an initiative. This statistic is particularly difficult to obtain accurately in medical management activities in which clinical returns are often not easily converted to financial equivalents. (See page 143, *An Understanding of Organizational Psychology*.)

2. *Balance sheets.* A balance sheet presents a financial picture of a company or organization at a fixed point in time (see Figure 4–1). As such, it is a "snapshot" that records the organization's assets, liabilities, and, in the case of a publicly owned company, the owner's equity. In its simplest form, the balance sheet provides a picture of how big the company is and how much of its size is owed to others. It typically presents several derivative statistics, often depicted as ratios (e.g., current ratio, quick ratio), that show how much and to what degree a company's assets and liabilities

Figure 4–1   Sample Balance Sheet

Balance Sheet: ABC Medical Corporation

Balance Sheet (as of December 31, 2004)

Assets

Current Assets

Cash	$ 50,000
Accounts Receivable	35,000
Total Current Assets	$ 85,000

Non-current Assets

Land	$200,000
Medical Office Building	1,579,000
Equipment (net of accumulated depreciation)	250,000
Total Non-current Assets	$2,029,000
Total Assets	**$2,114,000**

Liabilities and Shareholders' Equity

Current Liabilities

Accounts Payable to Suppliers	$ 25,000
Salaries Payable to Employees	32,000
Taxes Owed	52,000

Non-current Liabilities

Notes Payable to Lenders	$ 150,000
Total Liabilities	**$ 259,000**

Shareholders' Equity

Common Stock	$1,500,000
Retained Earnings	355,000
Total Shareholders' Equity	**$1,855,000**
Total Liabilities and Shareholders' Equity	**$2,114,000**

are committed to hard assets, outstanding loans, liabilities of other types, taxes, and other areas. The liquidity of the organization's assets, or the ability of the company to move cash, is an important part of this statement.

3. *Income statements.* Probably more important to managers than the financial statement or the balance sheet is the *income statement*, which is useful in the ongoing evaluation of a business or modeled initiative (see Figure 4–2). In the standard income statement, sources of revenue are listed at the top of the sheet, expenses are listed below in numerated "line item" form, and a "net income" is given at the bottom. This format is typically used to communicate the sales efforts of the organization and the costs that must be subtracted from profits.

Quality professionals should also consider the *accounting basis* when recording information in accounting ledgers. Many physicians or nurses initially entering hospital or managed care environments are used to the cash accounting, or *cash-basis accounting*, used in their practices. Here, revenue and costs are recognized in the month or period in which they occur. For a variety of reasons, large organizations follow *accrual-based accounting*, in which revenue and expenses may not match neatly within each month. In this approach, companies record revenue and expenses in the period in which they were incurred, regardless of the time in which money may have actually changed hands or in which a check was received. Accrual-based accounting requires regular upkeep of accounting ledgers but is more appropriate than cash-based accounting for organizations in which cash flows are not closely temporally linked.

In health care, real profitability and future growth are also assessed with *earnings before interest and taxes* (EBIT). This element is important in the income statements of both for-profit and not-for-profit health care companies because it identifies the "real" earnings of a company. The expanded concept of *earnings before interest, taxes, depreciation, and amortization* (EBITDA) is also often used in

Figure 4–2 Sample Income Statement

Income Statement: ABC Medical Corporation

Income Statement (for 2004)

Revenues

Patient Revenues	$ 1,575,000
Consulting Income	85,000
Investment Income	2,000
Total Revenues	**$ 1,662,000**

Expenses

Salary of Partners	853,347
Staff Wages	235,645
Laboratory Fees	32,583
Administrative Expenses	75,495
Interest Expense	3,453
Insurance	23,453
Total Expenses	**$ 1,223,976**
Net Income	**$ 438,024**

income statements when estimates of cash profitability are desired. Interest, taxes, depreciation, and amortization are used in financial and tax accounting to reduce taxable profits. Thus, EBIT and EBITDA represent earnings that are available for reinvestment in the company and are important in estimating profitability, the capital structure of the company, and other important concepts in both taxed and tax-exempt organizations.

4. *Statements of cash flows.* Another important accounting reporting tool is the *statement of cash flows* (see Figure 4–3). This statement typically shows the sources of cash received by the organization and provides an overview of whether or not the organization can move around liquid assets within its operations. This statement is typically of more interest to financial managers than to medical quality professionals, but its existence and general structure are worth reviewing.

The statement of cash flows accounts for the cash moving though the organization from operating, investing, and financing activities. Selling goods or services is the predominant method for realizing *operating cash flows*. The acquisition of non-current assets, particularly property and equipment, makes up the *investing* section of the statement and is needed for the company to function. Finally, the company's efforts to obtain cash for short- and long-term use are described in the *financing* section of the statement.

Statements of cash flows assess the effect of ongoing operations on the liquidity of the corporation and describe the relationships among the various components. The statement may reveal that the company is out of balance with respect to cash inflows and outflows, a situation that can precipitate a cash crisis, in which insufficient cash is available to meet the needs of the corporation. Alternatively, the statement may show the availability of too much cash, which suggests that the company is not making the best use of this resource.

5. *Annual reports.* A company's *annual report* is designed to provide an overview of the company and the company's financial position and is directed from the president to persons involved in run-

Figure 4–3   Sample Statement of Cash Flows

Cash Flows: ABC Medical Corporation

Statement of Cash Flows (for 2004)

Operations

Cash Flow from Operations	$ 1,662,000

Investing

Sale of Non-current Assets	0
Acquisition of Non-current Assets	–30, 000
Total Cash Flow from Investing	$ –30,000

Financing

Issue of Partner Stock	50,000
Dividends	–2,000
Total Cash Flow from Financing	$ 48,000

Net Change in Cash Flow	**$ 1,680,000**

ning the company, to stockholders, and to policyholders. The report typically contains annual and quarterly financial statements, including a balance sheet, an income statement, and a statement of cash flow, along with other information, such as a letter from the company president and a statement from an independent auditor. People who review these documents are often most interested in the supplementary information at the end of the report, particularly the "management letter" provided by the independent auditor. Areas of concern documented in the management letter may raise "red flags" among those concerned about the organization's assets and its future prospects of growth and performance

Types of Accounting Systems.

1. *Generally Accepted Accounting Principles.* Many of the accepted accounting principles in the United States have been developed through a centralized method called *generally accepted accounting principles* (GAAP). Annual reports, balance sheets, and similar types of accounting documents are all prepared using GAAP. These principles are set by general approval from three main formal organizations: the American Institute of Certified Public Accountants (AICPA), the Security and Exchange Commission (SEC), and the Financial Accounting Standards Board (FASB). These organizations gained influence in the development of accounting principles during the mid- to late 20th century. These accounting principles have not been adopted universally, however, and in many countries, different—sometimes completely different—accounting systems may be operating. Recently, several international organizations have sought to standardize financial accounting methods for use in international commerce.

2. *Statutory Accounting Standards.* Accounting and financial reporting can also include a variety of *statutory accounting standards* that are developed by government agencies. Statutory accounting principles are standardized, often on a national or state-by-state basis, and they are used by departments of health and departments of insurance to regulate health plans. Like income tax forms, these statutory forms contain a variety of financial and sometimes clinical or utilization information that is useful to the state or federal government. Statutory information may be calculated using certain algorithms that better allow state regulators to determine effectiveness, solvency, and similar aspects of health plan or hospital management.

The efforts of the National Association of Insurance Commissioners (NAIC) to develop "model acts" that outline standardized recommendations for writing legislative and statutory requirements have contributed significantly to generating order in the health care industry. Widespread adoption of these principles has helped develop a relatively consistent approach in the insurance industry across the country.

3. *Managerial Accounting.* In addition to offering financial accounting, business schools typically offer a course in *managerial accounting* that focuses more on the day-to-day workings of the corporation. The approaches used in managerial accounting are often not part of GAAP but are adopted regularly by organizations for internal use. The purpose of these approaches is to provide senior management with a clear view of financial events in the company.

An important concept in managerial accounting is *contribution income*, which is reflected in the *contribution income statement*. In this variation of the income statement, revenues and expenses are listed on a per-unit-of-production basis. Thus, the revenues from an individual "widget" are linked with expenses for that widget to show the *contribution margin*, or profit, from the sale of each widget. Fixed expenses or fixed overhead must also be taken into consideration, and these items are presented later in the contribution income statement. The value of this approach is that the overall profit can be calculated easily once the break-even point is known (i.e., the point at which the contribution margin from the sale of a certain number of widgets equals the amount of the fixed expenses or overhead). The application of this approach to medical management initiatives is clear. If a certain per-member per-month medical cost saving is anticipated from an intervention that costs a known amount, the number of individuals who need to be treated per month to cover the monthly—*or* overall cost—and overall fixed expenses of the initiative (the "break-even point") can be calculated. From these figures, the amount of profit from each additional member treated per month (the *marginal profit*) can be calculated.

In Box 4–4, the break-even point would occur when 23,000 members were treated; at this point, the revenues would equal the remaining expenses (that is, 23,000 members times the contribution

---

Box 4–4	Study Discussion and Example: Differences between a regular income statement and a contribution income statement

Standard income statements generally reflect sources of revenue and expenses, and then define the difference as net profit:

Form of a Regular Income Statement

Revenues	
Revenues	$ 100
Expenses	
Variable Expenses	$ 60
Fixed Expenses	$ 20
Profit (Loss)	**$ 20**

A contribution income statement presents variable revenues and expenses separately from fixed expenses and notes the relationship between the volume of business activity and the ultimate profitability of the organization.

Form of a Contribution Income Statement

	PMPY*	Total
Members Affected		50,000
Revenues		
Variable Revenues/Savings	$ 7	$350,000
Expenses		
Variable Expenses/Unit	$ –5	$250,000
Contribution Margin	$ 2	$100,000
Fixed Expenses		$46,000
Profit (Loss)		$54,000

*PMPY = Per member per year.

margin of $2 per member would generate $46,000, the amount needed to meet the fixed expenses). Above this point, the marginal profit of the effort would accrue at a rate of $2 per member per year.

A second important concept in managerial accounting is a relatively recent method of accounting called *activity-based cost accounting* (ABC) (see Table 4–3). In this approach, various sub-programs are broken out in the income statement and are represented separately in individually-identified revenue and expense categories. Various products might produce large or small amounts of revenue and thus generate large or small amounts of profit. This non-GAAP analysis allows managers to isolate solid performers or weaker performers in their product lines and to consolidate further these observations into an overall statement of effectiveness of their product development. In the case of clinical activities, this approach can be used to identify activities that yield or do not yield value or that have values with respect to each other. For example, one might sort out different activities that are worth keeping or discarding in a disease management program.

Accounting Skills Needed by Medical Managers.
All of the accounting tools described above are easily modeled on spreadsheets. The need for medical managers to develop the necessary skills to create financial models on spreadsheets cannot be overestimated. Using spreadsheets to create these models eases communications with other areas of the organization that are involved in financing and approving the budgets for clinical programs.[29] For example, activity-based cost accounting might allow medical managers to isolate various programs under their control and to separate the components for analysis. Such an approach is also useful in medical facilities that track individual doctors, medical groups, or facility locations.[30]

An overall understanding of financial accounting and formal financial statements is important for comprehending the state of an organization and the language of business. A working knowledge of managerial accounting is useful for communicating with people elsewhere in the organization. For example, medical managers must put together budgets that project anticipated costs for their organization. A medical manager who is not familiar with the various categories of cost in the budget—and the ways in which these costs can be modeled on spreadsheets—is at a clear disadvantage.

Other disadvantages of a lack of exposure to finance and accounting principles are subtler. For example, medical directors often report that the assigned office overhead or the percentage of the

Table 4–3	Example of Activity-Based Cost Accounting			
Product	**A**	**B**	**C**	**Total**
Revenue				
Variable Revenue	$50	$50	$20	$120
Expense				
Variable Expense	$30	$ 5	$ 5	$ 40
Fixed Expense	$15	$30	$ 5	$ 50
Profit (Loss)	$ 5	$15	$10	$ 30

organization's fixed expenses is high for their group. If the organization's *allocation strategy*, another concept in accounting for *internal cost transfers*, focuses on overall salary rather than head count, a group with higher salaries could be penalized by having to absorb a disproportionately higher share of office overhead. Medical managers who shun the study of finance as too threatening or too boring might not pick up such detail, and their ability to obtain funds for future organizational expansion may be affected. Similarly, requests by medical managers to increase staffing in a quality improvement department are often met with skepticism because solid accounting measures or business models to justify the expansion are lacking. Developing financial and accounting skills, or acquiring staff who have these skills, is becoming critical to the success of quality management departments.

Finance

As with economics and accounting, a lack of knowledge of the field of finance may put medical managers at a disadvantage and cause them to feel intimidated by managers with this knowledge. Medical managers should be familiar with common financial terms and how these terms are used in an organization, particularly if they are seeking to become recognized as legitimate managers in a large organization (see Appendix A at the end of this chapter). Financial concepts that medical managers need to understand are those surrounding the *cost of capital* and *discounted cash-flow analysis* as well as *budgeting*.

Costs of Capital.

Long- and short-term financial management decisions may be less applicable to junior or even senior medical managers than to financial managers. Nevertheless, medical managers must understand the effect of the cost of their department on the overall finances of the organization. The organization's finance officers are interested in the *expected rate of return* of various efforts by the organization. However, the expected rate of return is particularly difficult to calculate for medical initiatives that typically are not sold and that have only indirect relationships to changes in medical care costs. The effect of medical management activities often is not felt for many years, if at all, and the overall lack of certainty and precision complicates communication with financial managers trained to work with more precise terms.

Other communication difficulties may arise because medical managers do not comprehend the value of capital. Medical management staff members often do not appreciate, for example, that money used to fund various projects has a value of its own—that is, the value that it might achieve if it were invested in something else, even a bank account. The amount represents the *opportunity cost* that was sacrificed by using the money in one way as opposed to some other way. Aggressive valuation techniques subtract this amount from the ultimate return from a program to determine *economic value added* (EVA).[31] Incorporating these financial concepts when requesting additional funding for clinical activities is important for making a successful case to senior management.

Discounted Cash Flow Analyses.

Discounted cash flow analyses look at the time value of money. Briefly put, "money now is better than money later." For example, investing $100 at an interest rate of 8% will yield $108 in one year. Similarly, being owed $108 next year is the equivalent of being paid $100 now. The formula Future Value (FV) = Present Value (PV) times (1 + Interest Rate) creates a relationship that converts future cash or benefit into present dollars, in *net present value* calculations. Discounting future value in terms of present value in this way is frequently done in finance and is the accepted method used by financial officers to make those conversions. Familiarity with the correct use of this tool is important. Clinical managers often get into difficulty by trying to define more nebulous "quality gains" or "medical cost savings" in current economic terms. Incorrect use of the analysis, or faulty conclusions, can result.

Budgeting.

Working together on budgets is probably one of the most direct interactions that medical management staff has with financial staff. Senior managers unfamiliar with budgets frequently neglect the complicated, often tedious, spreadsheets and accounting statements required by other departments and underestimate the importance of these documents to the rest of the organization. As a result, the authority to prepare and interpret these documents is often yielded to persons with less commitment to understanding and managing clinical activities.

Budgets are prepared differently in nearly every organization but typically follow structures that are similar to the structure of the income statement (see Figure 4–2). Presented on a month-by-month basis and usually on spreadsheets, an entire year's expenses can be projected. The inability to follow a budget or to understand why individual budget categories are exceeded creates financing problems for senior management that in turn degrade medical managers' ability to function in an organization. Attention to budgets, while tedious, is a worthwhile exercise that should be undertaken by all medical managers, whether or not they are directly involved in the budgeting process.

Other General Business Principles

Medical managers need a general understanding of how the business community works. Knowing several concepts is extremely important in helping them interact with others in the organization. These concepts include:

1. Organizational planning and the planning process
2. Project management
3. Creation of business plans
4. Preparation of pro forma financial statements
5. Performance of sensitivity analyses
6. An understanding of organizational psychology

Organizational Planning and the Planning Process.

In health care organizations, considerable resources are often dedicated to planning. The importance of this process cannot be overstated. Effective planning ultimately results in creating a detailed project management plan for the organization that defines specific activities.

Planners often start by formulating an overall view of the purpose of the organization, called the *mission statement*. This statement is designed to identify the key reason for the organization's existence and is often limited to one or two sentences. Planners may also create a *vision statement* for the organization that provides an overview of the organization's goals, often with a bias of describing how the organization will fare under idealized circumstances. After planners define the organization's mission and vision, they often develop high-level goals, which outline how the organization will attain its mission. A statement of goals typically contains five or ten major elements around which the business will focus in the coming year. Each goal in turn has associated, measurable objectives that must be met by a specified time to ensure that the goal is reached. Project management grids typically identify each objective and outline key tactical steps needed to achieve the objectives. Thus, from the high-level mission statement, the organization's planners can define goals for achieving that mission as well as define specific tactics that will deliver the objectives within the year.

After planners have formulated goals and objectives, they typically move on to the detailed operational targets or achievable milestones that are listed in the management plan. Good managers usually name specific measures that indicate whether the plan is on track, and record them regularly. *Lag measures* inform planners retrospectively whether their goals have been achieved; examples are (1) records of net profits obtained after the corporation's books have been closed each month, and (2) patient satisfaction survey results. *Lead indicators*, which inform managers as to whether the corporation is on track in meeting a goal, are equally important; examples are (1) patient flow measures (e.g., new patient visits) as a means of assuring new patient flows, and (2) average daily collections, used to predict monthly earnings.

Project Management.

Project management becomes essential as the organization moves to ensure that the desired flow of information and direction is maintained throughout the year. Poorly managed organizations frequently fail to identify specific goals and objectives, and such organizations may spend considerable time in planning, without achieving tangible results. To be successful, clinical quality managers need training in project management and the ability to carry out the planning sequence. Several accreditation organizations, such as the NCQA, provide outlines for these types of planning processes as part of their required training. The leaders of these organizations have learned, as have many managers, that a well-thought-out and organized plan yields results when implemented effectively. Execution and results, not discussion or published articles, define success.

Good project management requires that all members of the initiative team understand their roles and responsibilities and know whether they are on track in executing the identified plan. Among the typical tasks of project management are identifying each key component of the project, identifying an accountable person to start the project, and setting an anticipated completion date. Simple grids, presented in a spreadsheet, can often be used in place of more expensive, formal project management programs, such as Microsoft Project.

Creation of Business Plans.

Successful business managers all report that a key to their success is the ability to plan and orchestrate a business initiative properly. Having a well-conceived business plan is frequently cited as a main factor for ensuring that an initiative is executed. Business plans can be created through many approaches, most of which have been published. An effective business plan is disciplined and focused, combining various components of the financial analysis to make the business case for proceeding with the initiative.

Key elements of a business plan, each typically described in a few paragraphs, include:

1. An overview of the industry or company and a description of any products that are being produced or are under consideration
2. An evaluation of the current market, including the advantages of the proposed initiative over competitors' initiatives
3. A formal outline of the proposed initiative and the opportunities that it provides the company
4. Marketing research that identifies the potential target market and the projected costs and revenues for the initiative
5. A formal design for implementing the initiative and a development schedule

| Box 4–5 | Exercise: Case analysis and problem for discussion |

Write a business plan that explains how a medical director of a health plan might request information from a disease management vendor as part of a request for proposal (RFP) for providing service as a vendor. Alternatively, explain how a medical director of a plan might use the business plan to justify a request of $4,000,000 to conduct a flu shot campaign in the community over a two-year period, and why you believe there would be a return on investment.

6. An overall operations plan that uses standard project management approaches
7. A profile of an accountable lead person and the credentials of the management and operations teams
8. An overview of the economics surrounding the business and the initiative including general profitability, sales potential, and so on
9. Anticipated risks and problems that could result in less-than-optimal outcomes
10. Financing arrangements and pro forma financial statements that outline return and costs over a period of several years
11. Estimated contracts, terms, agreements, and other items that must be negotiated
12. Exit strategy: the process for ending or discontinuing the program

The financial analysis, which need not be longer than five pages, may be presented in graphic or tabular form. Overall, the business plan should be a convincing statement that can be understood easily by a non-business partner. A business plan typically projects a financial loss in the first year or two of development and a profit in subsequent years. The reasons for the projected losses in the initial years are typically scrutinized carefully by financial managers to prevent the losses from persisting (see Box 4–5).

Preparation of Pro Forma Financial Statements.
Pro forma financial statements, which are typically part of a business plan, detail the financial cost and expenses of a project for several time periods in the future (see Figure 4–4). These statements generally identify cost savings and expenses for a project in each of the subsequent three years, and overall profitability and return on investment. Pro forma financial statements are used throughout the planning and financial processes to give financial managers an overview of the long-term effectiveness of a project. They are particularly useful when a project has high start-up costs and thus may appear to be financially untenable.

Performance Sensitivity Analyses.
In sensitivity analysis, which is often conducted with spreadsheets, the business project is modeled around a few initial key variables. A range of possible values for the variables is considered, and the effect on outcomes is noted. Sensitivity analyses allow managers to determine best- and worst-case outcomes of their undertaking, with respect to numbers of participants, financial return on investment, or other factors.

An Understanding of Organizational Psychology.
An important but often overlooked component in the business education of quality management professionals is the understanding of basic organizational psychology. This term refers to the com-

Figure 4–4 Example of a Pro Forma Financial Statement for a Planned Project

Estimated CHF QAPI Extra Payment Scanner Project Costs	2001 (July -December)	2002 (January - December)	2003 (January - December)	Total
Revenue:				
Minimum Extra Payment Potential		$375,000	$375,000	$750,000
Expenses:				
Staff:				
.5 FTE (Temporary RN) @ 19.80/hr	$9,652.50	$19,305.00	$19,305.00	$48,262.50
Onsite Expenses (e.g., travel, phone)	$2,000.00	$8,000.00	$8,000.00	$18,000.00
Hardware:				
Computer	$1,500.00			$1,500.00
Scuzi card	$85.00			$85.00
Scanner (Panasonic KDSS25D)	$2,500.00			$2,500.00
Software:				
Telform Single User License		$6,000.00		$6,000.00
Software Maintenance Agreement		$500.00	$500.00	$1,000.00
Mail: ($1.60/packet)				
Mailing Cost (983 initial packets)	$1,572.80			$1,572.80
Mailing Cost (1000/quarter)		$6,400.00	$6,400.00	$12,800.00
Envelopes (#793 – 1000/$64.80)	$64.60	$259.20	$259.20	$583.00
Printing:				
Paper (1000 sheets/$4.45)	$39.74	$22.91	$22.91	$85.56
Printing (0.6/sheet)	$5,362.80	$3,081.60	$3,081.60	$11,526.00
Total Expenses:	$22,777.44	$43,568.71	$37,568.71	$103,914.86
Net Revenues:	($22,777.44)	$331,431.29	$337,431.29	$646,085.14

The quality improvement department was asked to justify the purchase of a scanner and other equipment needed to send questionnaires to physicians about their congestive heart failure patients. The information gathered was to be used to apply for QAPI extra payment for conducting such a program.[32]

plex interaction of individuals in an organization and how these interactions advance or interfere with the organization's overall business direction. Senior managers often report that much of this knowledge is gained by experience.

Physician managers tend overall to adapt rather poorly to the complex social dynamics of larger organizations. Physicians are trained to operate as authority figures, not as equal team members with other staff. They become frustrated with the ease with which individuals in organizations can impede their progress or their projects. Several unpublished sources estimate the longevity of medical directors in their jobs to be 1.5 to 3 years.

Successful medical managers and chief medical officers have provided several recommendations to increase medical and clinical managers' effectiveness in working with nonmedical financial managers:[33]

1. Clinicians should strive to work in group environments. Physicians should develop experience working in teams performing administrative tasks. The autocratic, military model frequently used in hospitals, in which doctors are solidly in control, is less common in the business world.

2. Medical managers should relate to nonclinical financial managers on the financial managers' terms. Clinical managers should seek to make clinical concepts relevant to a layperson and should avoid using complex language or unfamiliar clinical terms.

3. When presenting to financial managers, clinical managers should underscore the financial effect of their activities, particularly when budgetary support is sought for what may be perceived as abstract clinical notions. For example, nonmedical managers may need to be educated about the financial value of increasing the rate of foot exams in people with diabetes.

4. Clinical managers should seek to identify with nonclinical managers. Effective steps might include: to cease wearing a white coat, to use lay terms as often as possible, and to obtain training in business and finance so as to appear less "alien" and more a part of the management team.

5. Clinical managers should prepare reports that are easily understood by people from varied backgrounds, and they should avoid complex journal-like presentations.

6. Clinical managers should study the motives and desires of senior managers and relate to them using the concepts described above.

The study of organizational psychology is beyond the scope of this chapter. Clinicians should note, however, that organizational psychology is frequently applied in health care corporations in a volatile circumstance—reorganization. Clinicians should also be aware that the organizational structure often develops along political lines.

Case Study for Discussion

The CEO of your company has made friends with the vice president of marketing of a national company that claims that it can provide case management effectively. The two have gone golfing, have had dinner together, and have had several "high-level" discussions about having the vendor replace some or all of your existing case management staff with the vendor's staff. Two of your senior vice presidents in totally unrelated areas concur that the vendor's proposal might be a viable option. The vendor claims that he can give your company an "eight to one return on investment," and will "guarantee" it.

You, the medical director, are now approached by the CEO, who admits that he might dissolve the case management area, but offers to give you 30 minutes to agree with his idea or talk him out of it. He is interested in the return on investment that you get *now*. What do you tell him? Your answer should address both an analytic approach using the principles of a financial analysis discussed above and recognition of the various political factors that may influence your choices.

Source: Fetterolf, AJMQ Jan/Feb 2003.

● Making the Business Case for Medical Quality

Thus far, we have presented an overview of the key business concepts that a quality manager must understand. A test application of this knowledge is to develop a program that will make the case for a quality management department. The program needs to address the practical questions that managers of quality departments are often asked by people seeking to adjust budgets and emphasis in the company, such as:

Can a business case be made for a quality management department?

What is the return on investment of quality management activities?

Should the number of quality department staff members be increased or decreased?

In answering such questions, properly applying the principles discussed in this chapter may make the difference between ongoing development and effectiveness of quality programs and a gradual erosion of departmental budgets.

Surprisingly, little has been written on how to develop the business case for quality management in a health plan.[33] Often, medical management presentations are not compelling, and medical directors and quality management professionals find themselves feeling marginalized or isolated from the rest of the management staff. Further, the approach to understanding the concept of medical management varies with one's perspective (society, payer, provider, patient), how one might identify costs and benefits (intangible, direct, medical, indirect, nonmedical, and so on), and the type of analysis one performs to determine whether medical management is effective.[5] Methods used to indirectly create value estimates for other business types can also be investigated.[34]

An analysis of the economic value of quality management at the departmental level should take into account the following factors:

1. *Government mandates.* In the United States, a virtual mandate for quality management programs in health care has been created by the government, forcing large organizations to pay attention to the issue of medical quality. The government has mandated these programs directly and also indirectly by specifying that external accrediting agencies be used. These external agencies hold back full accreditation unless certain quality programs and processes are in place, sometimes even specifying which ones are to be used. Such agencies include the Center for Medicare and Medicaid Services (CMS), the National Committee for Quality Assurance (NCQA), URAC, JCAHO, and local state departments of health and insurance, among others. This evolving "quality bureaucracy" has increased dramatically in size and complexity over the past several years. New programs are continually being added, existing programs are being expanded, and the linkages among the programs and various agencies and organizations are being forged at a pace that has been challenging for a single department in a managed care company or hospital to coordinate and oversee.

2. *Demands by the business community.* Recognizing the same issues as the government has, various payers in the business community (usually large employers) are also requiring or demanding participation in quality programs.

3. *Requirements for quality oversight.* Because current requirements for medical management and quality oversight are extensive, clinical management departments typically need to manage multiple programs and identify programs through their research that can be used to satisfy more than one criterion or standard at a time. Creating programs that have a competitive administrative over-

head structure necessitates being frugal with resources and using individual initiatives to handle multiple demands.

4. *Demands of business partners.* Various accounts or business partners may mandate the quality improvement activities of an organization. The need to comply with mandates is an effective argument for properly funding these activities, but it will not address the issue of whether resources are used most appropriately or efficiently by medical managers.

5. *Financial effect.* The financial effect of quality improvement activities on an organization is usually fairly small. Although the overall cost initially may seem high to financial managers, it can often be shown to be quite small on a per-member per-month basis in a health plan distributed across the entire membership. An effective strategy might be to compare the costs of quality management in health care with those of similar efforts in other industries.

6. *Trade-off between higher accreditation standard and lower cost.* The organization might develop several scenarios under which quality improvement programs could be increased or decreased. Decreasing these activities typically results in challenges from accreditation agencies, such as a reduction from an "excellent" to an "accredited" rating by the NCQA. Senior management will need to determine whether it is committed to the highest level of quality or whether it is willing to risk and tolerate a lower accreditation standard in exchange for a decreased cost to the organization.

7. *Results of estimates using mathematical tools.* The benefits of quality management activities in mathematical terms have been estimated using tools such as the NCQA quality dividend calculator, which is available on the NCQA website (*www.ncqa.org*).

8. *Social goals.* Finally, the goal of quality can be more than financial. The mission of an organization, the "desire to do the right thing," and the general pursuit of excellence are reasonable justifications for quality-related programs. Major employers are beginning to recognize the importance of employee satisfaction, productivity, and reduced absenteeism as goals in the delivery of health care.

Most health plan quality directors will eventually attempt to produce a comprehensive evaluation of quality management activities based on the above points. A comprehensive listing of the many demands made on an organization by various outside organizations creates a strong case for the existence of a single department to deal with them. Next, quality managers need to show that compliance-related quality improvement activities are carried out as efficiently as possible by comparing benchmarks with organizations of similar size and business scope, and demonstrating that multiple requirements are being addressed by each activity.

Justifying quality management activities at the level of an individual initiative often requires a different approach. Clinical initiatives frequently are multidimensional problems that have high variation and are nonlinear in scope. Clinical activities do not lend themselves to simple, "linear" approaches like the "return on investment" calculations one might do for a simple loan or business proposal. They have complex cost functions that change over time, and there are no standing accounting methods to present them to senior management; that is, there are no "generally accepted accounting procedures" available to discuss the financial impact of medical management initiatives.[35, 36]

Recently, as the total amount of money available for health care becomes increasingly limited, economists are working to determine the relative value of different interventions, in the form of *cost effectiveness analysis* (CEA). Developed in various ways, these efforts seek to combine both costs and clinical effectiveness in a single statistic or equation, to estimate the impact or "bang for the buck" from various clinical activities. If, for example, one has only a million dollars to spend on all clinical programs, the best allocation of scarce dollars can be guided by these methods.[37-43]

Quality management returns can be presented in economic terms by using a variety of methods: financial, clinical, social, and operational.

1. *Financial.* The benefit of a quality management initiative can be presented in terms of financial savings; for example, *hard dollar savings, soft dollar savings*, or *imputed savings*. Hard dollar savings are often most difficult to demonstrate because a specific amount of savings is predicted; for example, $1.50 saved for every $1.00 invested in an initiative. More typically, the benefit of an initiative is expressed in soft dollar savings, which are presented as a range in which the savings is likely to fall; for example, between $0.94 per dollar invested (a "negative return on investment") and $3.00 per dollar invested (with a likelihood of about $1.50 in savings per dollar invested). These typical ranges are often difficult for senior managers to accept, and considerable effort is needed to demonstrate that the dollar savings is positive. Imputed savings are more readily demonstrated because they are compiled from evidence in the literature. Here, a clinical background is useful because the quality manager identifies the return on investment from a multicenter, randomized, double-blind, placebo-controlled trial. For example, such a trial may show the return on investment in influenza vaccine to be $16.00 per dose of vaccine administered. By proposing that an additional 5,000 doses be administered through the hospital or plan program, the medical manager imputes that $80,000 in savings will accrue. Although convincing to a clinician, this evidence may be less so to a financial manager. The case can be strengthened by an analysis showing the change in influenza-related costs to the plan itself.

2. *Clinical methods.* The rationale for conducting quality improvement activities can also be explained in terms of clinical improvement in care. Clinical improvements are often difficult to describe in economic terms, however. For example, even though increasing the mammography rate is thought to reduce the progression to more complicated cancers and to increase the number of early cancers identified at the curative stage, its value for reducing medical care costs, or even saving individual lives, has not been established. The inability to establish a close link between the clinical activity and cost savings makes moving to "return on investment" logic difficult. Clinical improvement must be advanced on the basis of willingness to pay, an economic term used to describe the subjective estimation of valuation that accompanies making a purchase decision in the absence of a more rigorous accounting approach.[44] The lack of a clear path from clinical outcomes to the financial value of a clinical initiative makes budgeting difficult and puts senior management in the position of determining whether or not the clinical activity is worth the additional investment without a concrete method for doing so.[33, 45]

3. *Intangible or social methods.* Some reasons for undertaking quality management initiatives are unrelated to finances or clinical matters and instead have social value. This category of evaluation in the business plan also needs to be placed prominently in front of senior management. Intangible outcomes may include increased patient satisfaction, and perception in the market that the institution is on the "leading edge," which may have positive implications on sales. Again, these benefits fall into the "willingness to pay" category.[44]

4. *Operational methods.* The benefit of a quality management program can also be shown in terms of the ability of the program to deliver the program elements. Although this approach might first

be dismissed as purely a process—rather than an outcome—measure, the two have relevant points of overlap. In a disease management program, for example, the theory of the program may not be in doubt. Randomized, multicenter trials may have proven repeatedly that the elements of the program deliver value. For example, beta-blockers have been shown to help patients after a heart attack, and good diabetic control reduces long-term costs. What the program may need is the ability to deliver these elements to an entire population in a reasonable time, because taking several years to enroll a population, or enrolling only a fraction of the population, will not deliver value. Low or high operational performance in the implementation of a quality program or medical initiative is a quality indicator because failure to implement the program will produce no results.

In summary, quality managers must understand that the component pieces of quality management initiatives are often difficult to identify in financial terms but that a structured evaluation as part of the business value proposition is necessary to allow an appreciation of the initiative, by those evaluating the activity.

Recall that economics is not just about money but is about value and the movement of value within the organization and society. A senior executive may wish to know only whether or not it is "a red number or a black number." Directors or financing individuals may just want to know whether the number is "a big black number or a small black number" as part of the evaluation for assigning some level of funding. By being articulate in describing the process and the value in terms of financial, sales, marketing, or solid clinical results, an organization increases the likelihood of success in approved funding.

The Role of Government in Medical Management and Quality

In the United States, politics and government play a key role in paying for health care, in dispensing the amount and type of health care, in taxation, and in providing the definitions of benefits from the care provided. The political process is the ultimate arbiter acting through, or as an administrator of, federal, state, and local regulation.

Various aspects of health care have been a major focus of each new presidential administration. In the 1930s, with the Depression as a backdrop, the American Hospital Association embraced the Blue Cross/Blue Shield initiatives to pay for hospital confinements and admissions. Responsibility for health care began to move from the individual to groups, and in 1935 the Social Security Administration was established. World War II accelerated the move to increase fringe benefits in lieu of increasing wages, which had been frozen during the war. These events had the unintended consequence of making the government a partial payer, in as much as benefits are paid from pretax dollars. They also established the trend of insurance being linked to employment. The Hill-Burton Act of 1946 altered hospital financing by funding the construction of community hospitals, but it also mandated care for those unable to pay. Commercial insurers subsequently introduced the first dollar coverage of medical illness, which increased medical demand.

In the 1960s, the Health Providers Education Act of 1963 expanded medical education. The federal government (through Titles XVIII and XIX in 1965) formed the Medicare and Medicaid programs. This act was originally meant to create only a small program because the average American life expectancy at the time was only 67 years. The expectation was that only about two years of benefits would need to be funded. Instead, the act resulted in a program that now accounts for a major portion of governmental spending. The 1970s brought a federal exemption to state law for employers who assume more responsibility for their employees, the Employee Retirement and Income Security Act (ERISA) of 1974, as well as some efforts to standardize, improve, and possibly control the Medicare program with professional standards review organizations (PSROs).

Government efforts aimed at cost-shifting, managing physician practices, cost-containment, the development of practice guidelines, and the emergence of evidence-based medicine have been documented throughout the past two decades. During the 1990s, an excess of hospital beds developed because the cost of all building and other capital improvements could now be directly passed back to the government. Virtually no aspect of the American health care system has been immune to governmental experimentation and intervention. In some cases, these efforts have involved micro-management, such as the Tax Equity and Fiscal Responsibility Act (TEFRA) in Medicare, risk contracting, Medicare Choice programs, Medicare preferred provider organizations (PPOs), federal government demonstration programs, and efforts of the Centers for Medicare and Medicaid Services (CMS, formerly the Health Care Financing Administration, HCFA) and its subcontractors. Medicare Part D regulations created in 2003 and 2004 extend this influence into pharmacy regulation as well. Since the mid-1990s, the federal government has required Medicare and Medicaid to adopt the Quality Improvement Standards for Managed Care (QISMIC). Similarly, states have required the participation of their Medicaid programs. In some cases, the states have provided the experimental grounds for innovations, new programs, and financing incentives, many of which have eventually been implemented on a national level.

Case Study and Discussion Questions

Medical costs for a health plan have been increasing over the past several years. The plan actuaries predict a flattening in the trend because costs "can't keep getting higher." They also note that economic analyses by the federal government (in a CMS report) suggest considerable debate about the leveling of costs in the near future. They admit that "provider reform" efforts by the federal government to control costs are doomed to failure, and that costs could keep going up. The consequences for the local economy are already being noted by the health plan's accountants, who report that increases in regional health care costs are causing them to consider moving business out of the region or even overseas, where health care costs are more moderate.

The chief medical officer is asked to comment. She notes that costs are up in every category. She also notes that various classes of emerging technologies continue to arrive in increasing numbers, and that the demographics of the plan suggest that the aging population will continue to have a great effect on cost. The vice president of provider relations observes that vertical and horizontal market consolidation in the area, as well as declining hospital margins, will make it unlikely that simple price controls will be effective because reimbursements to hospitals may need to go up this year. He admits that providers also have not had a fee increase for some time, are being hit with rising malpractice premiums, and are unlikely to settle for any reduction in fees. He concedes that physicians may be leaving the state because of low reimbursement and high malpractice premiums and that Medicare recently had to retreat from a planned reduction in physician payment. In his view, multiple economic factors seem to point to continuously increasing costs. The group concludes that the percentage of the gross national product attributed to health care, now edging to 14%, will rise even higher. These national trends are likely to be reflected in local health plans as well as in cost drivers.

The chief medical officer is asked to participate in a workgroup that will "brainstorm" methods of cost control. Several managers believe that cutting payments to physicians is the only way to reduce consumption of medical services. Others argue that better management of individuals will be the most cost-effective method. Still others maintain that the days of managed care are over, and that real cost savings will come through reducing unnecessary variation by applying quality tools.

What should the chief medical officer's advice to the group be? In formulating an answer, consider the following questions in light of the contents of this chapter:

1. What economic forces in the early 21st century make the solution to this problem so difficult?

2. How might a health care organization plan for various changes that are likely to come from governmental concern about the issue?

3. Will the economic power of physicians in highly concentrated markets increase or diminish as a result of these changes? How will this increase or decrease affect physicians' power in negotiations with the plan?

4. How might physicians change their planning processes?

Case Study

The Evolution of Laws Dealing with Health Care in Pennsylvania

During the past 10 years, Pennsylvania has seen an explosion of legislation aimed at defining, administering, mandating, and directing health care services in the state. The focus of the legislation began by determining specific answers to simple questions, such as "Who is a doctor?" or "Who is a dentist?" As time advanced, new types of practitioners were defined, as was the scope of their practices. Payment demands from these practitioners led to legislation that included them in the range of insured services, sometimes mandating their inclusion. Legislators have also addressed what can and cannot be covered among benefits, even mandating specific items, such as coverage for items needed to treat diabetes. Laws have sought to first define, and then limit, managed care activities, and to control the practice of selling insurance for health benefits. Examples of recently enacted laws that specifically address the quality of care are listed in Appendix B. Recent concerns about privacy have led to extensive legislative and regulatory treatises on what is and is not personal information, who can or cannot receive it, and what the consequences of noncompliance might be. Certain diagnoses—psychiatric conditions, drug and alcohol abuse, and AIDS—have special status, and certain rules surround their disclosure. The list of legislated topics continues to develop and expand. Some of the more representative recent legislative changes are noted in Appendix B.

The significance of these changes on quality professionals is clear. An increasing need to be cognizant of what can and cannot be done, and of what must and must not be done, defines the quality professional role as one of compliance officer as well as clinician.

The Reagan administration, beginning in 1981, passed budget reconciliation acts that changed the way health care in general, and Medicare in particular, is administered. The Tax Equity and Fiscal Responsibility Act (TEFRA) of 1982 provided for Medicare risk contracting, and the Comprehensive Omnibus Budget Reconciliation Act (COBRA) of 1985 affected health insurance by removing the requirement that made continuous employment a prerequisite for health plan coverage. The Omnibus Budget Reconciliation Act (OBRA) of 1987 enhanced the quality of life for nursing home residents; OBRA of 1989 introduced a fee schedule for physicians based on a relative-value schedule; and OBRA of 1990 brought in anti-dumping laws for hospital emergency rooms. Other key acts included the Health Care Quality Improvement Act of 1986, the Balanced Budget Act (often referred to as the "BBA"), and the Emergency Medical Treatment and Active Labor Act (EMTALA).

In 1993, during the Clinton administration, the burgeoning costs of health care were of such concern that First Lady Hillary Rodham Clinton was appointed to develop a national health plan. More than 100 academics, consultants, and government officials were "squirreled away" in the Old Executive Office building, where they developed the Health Security Act for the 103rd Congress of 1993, a 1,342-page document that aimed ". . . to ensure individual and family health care coverage for all Americans in a manner that contains the rate of the growth in health care costs and promotes responsible health insurance practices, to promote choice in health care, and to ensure and protect the health care of all Americans." The act, according to President Clinton, was grounded in six basic principles: security, simplicity, savings, quality, choice, and responsibility. By design, this working group included no representatives of the medical practice or medical business communities.

Although the Health Security Act ultimately did not pass, many states received the message that the federal government could—and would—make health care a federal issue and was willing to pre-empt states' rights if necessary. Immediately thereafter, the process started at state levels, where legislation, regulation, and rules could be applied to the problems of access, cost, and quality. The nation is currently in a cycle in which the balance of cost, quality, and access is altering because of individual concerns about health care expenditures, quality, patient safety, and access to health care.

The role of government in the health care delivery system has been expanding over time but lately has exploded as financing, demand, and emotion collide over many key issues. Legislative action has increased impressively over the past decade, and the number and reach of bills increase each year. Legislatures have sought to mandate benefits, reduce the control of managed care, alter funding mechanisms, and shift accountabilities. A list of legislative activities as they affect the marketplace in one state (Pennsylvania) is shown in Appendix B. A review of the breadth and scope of the legislation and the attendant regulatory environment demonstrates this trend.

As we enter the 21st century, the United States is confronting a recurrence of exploding health care costs, with double-digit inflation in commercial and governmental programs. Concerns are rising that efforts to control medical costs on the provider and insurer side are failing, and that the nation will enter a critical period in 10 years. Interim steps will include more employee cost shifting, efforts to adjust "demand management," and variations on medical management designed to decrease costs. Demand management refers to efforts designed to control the use of medical services by the patients themselves, such as providing patient education as a means of lowering overuse of ER services for minor care. The forces driving medical costs, however, are felt by many to be insensitive to these measures, and concern is growing that government intervention will be necessary. Because interventions in a crisis will, for the most part, be unpalatable to the general public (e.g., rationing, limited access, reduced payments, limited end-of-life care), one might anticipate that these measures will not be proposed until late in the course of the crisis.

Health Care as a Public Good

A key component in providing health care is the dual consideration of where the resources come from and how important it is that they be used for health care. Society must provide the answers, which will affect practitioners, companies that supply the medications, medical equipment, health care facilities, and other parts of the administrative infrastructure that are necessary wherever patients are being treated. Finance, economics, and government, in the form of politics and policy, will determine the final form of these answers.

A basic issue must be resolved before this debate can even take place. As discussed on a more simplistic level, economics and policy are ultimately systems for allocating limited resources. Allocation decisions can be made effectively only if the various demands for resources can be ranked in importance. Many factors affect these rankings, including the values and goals of the society and who will make the allocation decisions. Health care has been tested severely in the marketplace and in the press over the past several decades, in part because of our health care system's increased ability to affect health status.

From the standpoint of pure inputs and outputs, a society wants a healthy and happy populace that will be productive and at the same time consume goods and services. Both factors support the capitalistic system. Two major movements in medical quality directed to this end are demand management and case management. These movements are fledgling efforts to better match resources to need, and to achieve better output as a result. To begin to consider the optimal allocation of health resources, we must first define what health is. Is it simply the lack of disease, or does it mean a basic level of functioning? Along with this consideration is the question of what falls under the purview of health care. Are these health care problems or social problems? Should we consider these issues when we determine what to spend currently and in the future for the care of our citizens? A bigger question is, "How much health care is enough?" Is prevention important, or will we continue to have a rescue mentality, waiting until patients are sick before we intervene? Along with this consideration, we must ask, "How much personal responsibility should individuals take with regard to their health behaviors?" New questions arise about where treatment ends and enhancement begins. As we understand better the basic processes of biology, physiology, and genetics, and as our technical skills improve, we will build on our current crude ability to actually increase the performance of the human organism. Then the question will not simply be who receives the treatment but also whether these procedures should be allowed at all.

Another key concept that emphasizes the difficulty of providing quality medical care is that of risk. Health and sickness are the products of multiple factors, including genetic makeup, preventive maintenance, and environmental factors. The first is the result of the genetic lottery (i.e., "pick your parents wisely"). The second is a psychosocial—and to some degree an economic—factor, in which the individual and society have some input. The last is a result of probabilities; that is, certain things will happen as a result of at least some randomness. Health is paid for by insurance because of the unequal burden that these factors place on different individuals. Insurance spreads around the risk and the cost of illness. The cost is distributed over a population and for the individual over time. There are some problems with this method. One is the problem of adverse selection. The insurance company seeks to have a customer population that uses as few resources as possible. It accomplishes this goal through selection mechanisms, such as eliminating coverage for preexisting conditions, setting up procedures that exclude the sicker patients, and other underwriting practices. In turn, insurance spokespersons often claim that nuances of insurance regulations and business requirements may cause the sicker patients to choose one plan over another, thereby increasing use and cost. "Adverse selection" or the statistical movement of healthy patients away from an insurer to a competitor can be created by a number of subtle and not so subtle practices that operate in the environment of complex regulation. Adverse selection, over time, can result in a nonprofitable position for an insurer, who must return investment to those who have supported the organization (if a stock corporation) or at least cause it to break even (if not-for-profit).

Public policy is a mixture of the private market and the public sector. The government becomes involved in a process when there is a market failure; that is, when the market fails to match supply and demand properly. Health is again unusual, in that the presence of insurance to some degree increases the demand for health care. Also, a dissymmetry of information with regard to provider, process, and other factors tends to work against the consumer.

Insurance companies report that the major ways to deliver financial value are through risk pool management and contracting. Risk pool management occurs regularly with experience rated programs. Eliminating risky members, or weighting heavily in favor of healthy members (called cherry picking), can substantially lower overall health care costs and insurance premiums. Risk pools can be managed in a variety of subtle ways. High-deductible plans can discourage both health care use and the enrollment of sicker members. Similarly, predatory pricing of provider services in certain markets can bring a lower price at the expense of physician salaries. As a large purchaser of services, the federal government in the Medicare program can demand and obtain lower doctors' fees in this manner. As health care costs continue to rise, these types of maneuvers are being observed in many markets and in various forms. If ill patients are becoming disenfranchised, and doctors are being pressured to operate at increasingly lower levels of reimbursement, the all-important question becomes, "Where might these trends lead?"

Case Study

Economic Approach to Scarce Resources

A new, artificial liver has been a great success. It improves liver function in those lucky enough to have access to it, to the point that they are able to return to their maximum level of life activity. However, it does not totally cleanse the body of the destructive hepatitis virus, and therefore people who use it must stay on it permanently to continue receiving benefits. Patients are electing to do this instead of receiving a transplant. The machine generates much toxic waste and requires a filter that, so far, can only be made from platinum; the filter cannot be reused for four days because of extensive cleansing and refitting procedures.

The search for an effective hepatitis vaccine has been hampered by a lack of funding. The question now is, "How can more of the people afflicted with the hepatitis virus be given access to the machine; or should the priority be to develop vaccines, increased transplantation abilities, or both?" Should such efforts be funded through private insurance, or through a government program? Many of those afflicted are younger, and a number have drug problems and other diseases. A great deal of active lobbying to do something soon on the part of those already infected has occurred.

Many states have lagged behind in their efforts because the disease is linked to drug use and sexual contact. These states have opted for a prevention program based on abstinence and have steadfastly resisted any attempts to otherwise handle the disease and the new treatments.

The following questions are among those confronted by medical quality practitioners:

1. Which policy alternatives should be considered in addressing this problem?
2. Which economic questions must be addressed to evaluate these alternatives?
3. How can the medical quality practitioner help evaluate these alternatives?
4. What external issues could arise as a result of the various policy alternatives?
5. What considerations enter into how such an artificial liver service would be priced? Does the problem lend itself more to a public or to a private solution?

The following are some general guidelines about the case:

- The major options include: (1) doing nothing; (2) having industry further develop the artificial liver machine and having costs covered under private insurance; (3) funding the development of a vaccine instead; (4) increasing the transplant capability; and (5) starting a nationwide, federally-funded program that gives access to all applicants.
- The cost of the various programs must be considered. Even the alternative of "doing nothing" has costs, because it may mean that more patients receive disability payments or become wards of the state. Important questions include: Where is the money to come from, and how will it be raised? Are there ways in which a public-private partnership can evolve? What are the costs? What other programs might suffer as a result of the new program?
- Medical quality practitioners can use process-improvement and new technology assessment techniques to evaluate the various alternatives. They can also determine whether other parts of the process might benefit from evaluation.
- One obvious external issue is the effect on the environment from the toxic wastes. Will this factor make it difficult to place the clinics? Another issue is the economic impact of this program. Will it increase reckless behaviors in the young, as some conservatives predict?
- The pricing of such a service must include the actual cost of material, the cost of services, the cost of research and development, and the cost of disposing of generated materials, among others. If the private sector is involved, pricing must also include profits and a mechanism to repay any capital outlay costs. As in most situations, reasons for the government to take the lead are mixed. If the demand is not high enough to allow profits to be made, the investor will be reluctant to fund the effort. If it is controversial, a national stance may be necessary to overcome resistance.

Conclusion

Economics, finance, and accounting principles developed in the business community have a pervasive influence that cannot be ignored by contemporary clinical quality managers. The rapid expansion of the health care infrastructure over the past 30 years has required and driven an increasingly business-oriented focus to these clinical matters. As health care cost controls fail, and the ability of the private sector to regulate costs and quality falters, increasing governmental intervention can be expected. In a sense, there is no right answer to the optimal way to spend health care resources. At the societal level, optimal use of resources means directing testing and services to those most likely to benefit from the intervention. At the individual level, the issue is more one of a two-person, zero-sum game, where whenever the system wins, the individual perceives that he or she has lost, and vice versa. Quality professionals must work within the margin, seeking to define what is of high value, what is essential, and what will yield the best results.

Appendix A

Study List: Terms and Acronyms Used

accounting basis
accrual basis of accounting
activity-based cost accounting
AHRQ (Agency for Healthcare Research and Quality) annual report
BBA (Balanced Budget Act)
balance sheet
break-even point
budget process
business plan
business sensitivity analysis
CAHPS (Consumer Assessment for Health Plans Study)
CAQH (Council for Affordable Quality Healthcare)
cash basis of accounting
cash crisis
cherry picking
CMS (Center for Medicare and Medicaid Services)
contribution income statement
contribution margin
cost of capital
CQI (continuous quality improvement)
current ratio
discounted cash flow
earnings per share
ERISA (Employee Retirement and Income Security Act)
EVA (economic value added)
expected rate of return
experience rated
FACCT (Foundation for Accountability)

FASB (Financial Accounting Standards Board)

financial accounting

GAAP (Generally Accepted Accounting Principles) hard dollar savings

HEDIS (Health Plan Employer Data and Information Set)

highly concentrated markets

Hill-Burton Act

hospital physician joint venture

income statement

intangible savings

integrated delivery system

internal cost transfer

JCAHO (Joint Commission on the Accreditation of Healthcare Organizations)

lag measures

lead measures

macroeconomics

management letter

managerial accounting

marginal profit

microeconomics

mission statement

monopoly

monopsony

NCQA (National Committee for Quality Assurance)

net present value calculation

OBRA (Omnibus Budget Reconciliation Act)

operating, investing, and financing activities

price elasticity of demand

price taker

pro forma statements

project management

QISMC (Quality Improvement Standards for Managed Care)

quality assurance

quick ratio

return on assets

return on equity

return on investment

soft dollar savings

statement of cash flows

statistical quality control

statutory accounting models

TEFRA (Tax Equity and Fiscal Responsibility Act)

URAC (currently DBA as "American Accreditation HealthCare Commission")

willingness to pay

⬤ Appendix B

Legislative Actions That Affect Health Plans in One State (Pennsylvania)

(Prepared by Highmark Government Affairs Department in Highmark, Inc.)

Act or Public Law:	Description:
PA *Act 35 of 1992*	Effective November 1992, Act 35 requires all group and individual policies to provide coverage for childhood immunizations.
PA *Act 148 of 1992*	Effective February 1993, Act 148 requires all group and individual insurance policies to cover mammography screening for women age 40 and over and with any mammogram based on a physician's recommendation for women under 40.
PA *Act 20 of 1994*	Effective June 1994, Act 20 requires all insurers to include in all group and individual policies coverage for an annual screening pap smear and gynecological exam for women.
PA *Act 15 of 1996*	Effective immediately, Act 15 requires the Department of Health to establish a statewide program for the prevention of Hepatitis B through the immunization of children. This includes having Hepatitis B placed on the list of diseases that require immunization for entry into school after August 1, 1997.
PA *Act 112 of 1996*	Effective January 1997, Act 112 requires insurers to reimburse an insured or provider for medically necessary services performed in a hospital emergency facility due to a medical emergency. Act 112 defines a "medical emergency" as: a medical condition with acute symptoms of severity or severe pain for certain conditions.
Health Insurance Portability and Accountability Act (HIPAA) of 1996 P.L. 104-191	HIPAA institutes insurance market reforms by guaranteeing the availability and renewability of health insurance coverage for certain employees and individuals. HIPAA also establishes benefits parity for mental health benefits and minimums for maternity and newborn lengths of stay (outlined below). Requires insurers to accept all group applicants; Prohibits preexisting condition exclusions—conditions for which medical advice, diagnosis, care or treatment was recommended or received in the 6-month period prior to the enrollment date—for a period in excess of 12 months (18 months for late enrollees). May not impose pre-existing condition exclusions on certain newborns, adopted children or pregnant women; Prohibits discrimination based on health status, medical condition, claims experience, receipt of health care, medical history, genetic information, evidence of insurability (including conditions arising out of acts of domestic violence), or disability; Establishes a four-year demonstration project to give tax-preferred status to medical savings accounts when accompanied by a high-deductible health insurance policy.

Act or Public Law:	*Description:*
PA *Act 191 of 1996*	Effective June 20, 1997, Act 191 requires all individual and group health insurance policies that provide prescription drug benefits to include coverage for the cost of medically necessary nutritional supplements for the therapeutic treatment of phenylketonuria, galactosemia, and homocystinuria if administered under the direction of a physician.
PA *Act 4 of 1998*	Effective March 29, 1998, Act 4 prohibits employers from terminating or disciplining an employee who fails to report to work due to the closure of roads during a state of emergency that has been declared by the Governor. The bill exempts police, emergency service personnel, hospital and nursing home staffs; essential health care professionals; public utility personnel; oil and milk delivery employees, and radio and television personnel.
PA *Act 19 of 1998*	Effective February 18, 1998, section 5704 of Act 19 affects personnel of businesses engaged in telephone marketing or telephone customer service by means of wire, oral, or electronic communication to intercept such marketing or customer service communications where such interception is made for the sole purpose of training, quality control, or monitoring by the business, provided that one party involved in the communications has consented to such intercept. Any communications recorded pursuant to this paragraph may only be used by the business for the purpose of training or quality control. Unless otherwise required by federal or state law, communications recorded pursuant to this paragraph shall be destroyed in one year from the date of recording.
PA *Act 26 of 1998*	Effective April 18, 1998, Act 26 establishes charges for copies of medical records, particularly for legal cases where records are subpoenaed.
PA *Act 98 of 1998*	Effective February 12, 1999, Act 98 will require individual and group health insurance policies to provide coverage for diabetic supplies and related education. Specifics of Act 98 include: Except to the extent that the benefits are already covered under another policy, individual and group health plans must provide coverage for diabetic equipment and supplies (blood glucose monitors and supplies, insulin, injection aids, syringes, certain orthotics, etc.).
Mammography Quality Standards Reauthorization Act of 1998—HR 4382 (P.L. 105-248)	P.L. 105-248 (HR 4382) re-authorizes the Mammography Quality Standards Act of 1992. The law states that any facility that performs any mammogram shall maintain the mammogram in the permanent medical records of the patient for a period of not less than 5 years or not less than 10 years if no subsequent mammograms of such patient are performed at the facility, or longer if mandated by state law. The law also affords patients with direct notification of mammogram test results in terms they can understand.
Omnibus Consolidated and Emergency Supplemental Appropriations Act of 1998—(HR 4328) (P.L. 105-277), Cont.	P.L. 105-277 also includes the **Women's Health and Cancer Rights Act of 1998**, which requires all group health plans and health insurance issuers in the individual market that cover mastectomies to cover reconstructive surgery on the breast affected by mastectomy and surgery and reconstruction of the unaffected breast to produce symmetrical appearance. Prostheses and physical complications in all stages of mastectomy, including lymphedemas, are also covered. Treatment shall be determined in consultation with the attending physician and the patient. The coverage may be subject to annual deductibles and coinsurance provisions. Finally, the bill states that written notice of the coverage must be delivered to health plan consumers on enrollment and annually thereafter; but not later than January 1, 1999.

Act or Public Law:	Description:
PA *Act 150 of 1998*	Act 150 would require insurers to provide coverage for mental health benefits to all groups with 50 or more employees, effective April 19, 1999. Briefly, Act 150 does the following: The bill covers serious mental illnesses as defined by the American Psychiatric Association, including schizophrenia, bipolar disorder, obsessive-compulsive disorder, major depressive disorder, panic disorder, anorexia nervosa, bulimia nervosa, schizo-affective disorder, and delusional disorder; however, it does not include drug or alcohol abuse.
PA *Act 89 of 2001*	Effective February 28, 2002, Act 89, the Infant Hearing Education, Assessment, Reporting, and Referral Program requires the Department of Health to establish a program for hospitals to screen all newborns for hearing loss before leaving the hospital, in addition to providing information, instructions to parents for follow-up care.
PA *Act 81 of 2002*	Effective June 28, 2002, Act 81 of 2002 brings Pennsylvania into compliance with the Women's Health and Cancer Rights Act of 1998 by removing language in Act 51 of 1997 that set a six-year limit on when a woman could have reconstructive surgery following a mastectomy. The act also establishes notification requirements at enrollment and on an annual basis; clarifies coverage for all "physical complications" following a mastectomy; and prohibits insurers from denying to a patient eligibility or continued eligibility to enroll or renew coverage under the terms of the health insurance policy solely for the purpose of avoiding the requirements of the act.
PA *Act 83 of 2002*	Effective August 28, 2002, Act 83, the College and University Student Vaccination Act requires university and college students to receive a one-time vaccination against meningococcal disease before residing in a dormitory or housing unit. Exemptions are allowed for religious or other reasons if the college provides detailed information about the risks associated with meningitis and the availability and effectiveness of the vaccine.
PA *Act 135 of 2002*	Effective December 25, 2002, Act 135 of 2002 amends the Dental Law to establish standards and minimum educational requirements for the administration of general anesthesia in dentists' offices.

References

1. Couch JB. *Health Care Quality Management for the 21st Century.* Tampa, FL: Hillsboro Printing Co. for the American College of Physician Executives; 1991.

2. Crosby P. *Quality Is Free.* New York, NY: New American Library; 1979.

3. Crosby P. *Quality Without Tears.* New York, NY: McGraw-Hill Book Company; 1984.

4. Donabedian A. *Explorations in Quality Assessment and Monitoring. Volume II. The Criteria and Standards of Quality.* Ann Arbor, MI: Health Administration Press; 1982.

5. Eisenberg J. Clinical economics. A guide to the economic analysis of clinical practices. *JAMA.* November 24, 1989;262(20):2879–2886.

6. McLaughlin C, Kaluzny A. *Continuous Quality Improvement in Healthcare.* Gaithersburg, MD: Aspen Publishers; 1999.

7. Walton M. *The Deming Management Method.* New York, NY: Perigee Books; 1986.

8. Gold M. *Cost Effectiveness in Health and Medicine.* Report of the U.S. Public Health Service Panel on Cost Effectiveness in Health and Medicine. Oxford University Press; 1996.

9. Berwick D. *Curing Health Care. New Strategies for Quality Improvement.* San Francisco, CA: Jossey-Bass; 1990.

10. Drummond M, O'Brien B, Stoddart G, Torrance G. *Methods for the Evaluation of Health Care Programmes,* 2nd ed. New York, NY: Oxford Medical Publications; 1998.

11. Drummond M, McGuire A. *Economic Evaluation in Health Care: Merging Theory with Practice.* New York, NY, and Oxford, England: Oxford University Press; 2001.

12. Corrigan J, Greiner A, Erickson S. *Fostering Rapid Advances in Health Care: Learning From System Demonstrations.* Washington, DC: National Academy Press; 2002.

13. Kohn L, Corrigan J, Donaldson M. *To Err Is Human—Building a Safer Health System.* Washington, DC: National Academy Press; 1999:1–13.

14. National Academy of Sciences. Priority areas for national action: Transforming health care quality 2003. 2003.

15. Millenson M. *America's Health Care Challenge: Rising Costs.* A report commissioned by the American Association of Health Plans. Washington, DC: AAHP. January 22, 2002.

16. Montgomery D. *Introduction to Statistical Quality Control.* 3rd ed. New York, NY: John Wiley and Sons; 1997.

17. Carey R, Lloyd R. *Measuring Quality Improvement in Healthcare.* New York, NY: Quality Resources, 1995.

18. Langley P. Is cost effectiveness modeling useful? *The American Journal of Managed Care.* February 2000;6 (2):250–251.

19. Coddington D. *Making Integrated Health Care Work.* Englewood, CO: Center for Research in Ambulatory Health Care Administration; 1996.

20. Centers for Medicare and Medicaid Services. *Health Care Industry Market Update. Managed Care.* Washington, DC: Centers for Medicare and Medicaid Services. March 24, 2003.

21. Dornbursch R, Fischer S. *Macroeconomics.* 5th ed. New York, NY: McGraw-Hill; 1990.

22. Jacobs P. *The Economics of Health and Medical Care.* Gaithersburg, MD: Aspen Publishers; 1996.

23. Scherer FM, Ross D. *Industrial Market Structure and Economic Performance.* 3rd ed. Dallas, TX: Houghton Mifflin; 1990.

24. Mansfield E. *Economics.* 6th ed. New York, NY: W.W. Norton; 1989.

25. Wessels WJ. *Economics.* New York, NY: Barron's Business Review Series; 1993.

26. Taylor T. Economics (Part I and Part II) Audio Tape Course. The Learning Company, Inc.; 1996.

27. Phelps C. *Health Economics.* New York, NY: Addison-Wesley; 1997.

28. Santerre R, Neun S. *Health Economics: Theories, Insights, and Industry Studies.* Chicago, IL: Irwin; 1996.

29. Kaplan R, Cooper R. *Cost and Effect: Using Integrated Cost Systems to Drive Profitability and Performance.* Boston, MA: Harvard Business School Press; 1998.

30. Baker J. *Activity-Based Costing and Activity-Based Management for Health Care.* Gaithersburg, MD: Aspen Publishers; 1998.

31. Hubbell W. Combining economic value added and activity based management. *Journal of Cost Management.* Spring 1996:18–29.

32. Gladowski P, Fetterolf D, Beals S, Holleran MK, Reich S. Analysis of a large cohort of HMO patients with congestive heart failure. *American Journal of Medical Quality.* April 2003;18(2):73–81.

33. Fetterolf D. Commentary: Presenting the value of medical quality to nonclinical senior management and boards of directors. *American Journal of Medical Quality.* Jan/Feb 2003;18(1):10–14.

34. Luehrman T. What's it worth? A general manager's guide to valuation. *Harvard Business Review.* May-June 1997:132–142.

35. Plocher D, Brody R. Disease management and return on investment. In: Kongstvedt PR, Plocher D, eds. *Best Practices in Medical Management.* Sudbury, MA: Jones & Bartlett; 1998:397–406.

36. NCQA. *The Business Case for Health Care Quality. www.ncqa.org/somc2001/bizcase/somc_2001_biz_case.html* Accessed Jan 2002.

37. Blissenbach H. Use of cost-consequence models in managed care. *Pharmacotherapy.* 1995;15(5):59s–61s.

38. Clancy C, Kamerow D. Evidence-based medicine meets cost-effectiveness analysis. *JAMA*. July 24/31, 1996;276(4):329–330.

39. Galvin R. The business case for quality. Developing a business case for quality will require a deliberate approach, with all economic parties at the table. *Health Affairs*. Nov/Dec 2001:57–58.

40. Haddix A, Teutsch S, Shaffer P, et al. *Prevention Effectiveness: A Guide to Decision Analysis and Economic Evaluation*. New York, NY, and Oxford, England: Oxford University Press; 1996.

41. Litvak E, Long M, Schwartz S. Cost-effectiveness analysis under managed care: Not yet ready for prime time? *The American Journal of Managed Care*. February 2000;6(2):254–256.

42. Torrance G. Preferences for health outcomes and cost-utility analysis. *The American Journal of Managed Care*. 1997;(Suppl 3):S8–S20.

43. Weinstein M, Siegel J, Gold M, et al. Recommendations of the panel on cost-effectiveness in health and medicine. *JAMA*. October 16, 1996;276(15):1253–1258.

44. Gafni A. Willingness to pay in the context of an economic evaluation of healthcare programs: Theory and practice. *Am. J. Man. Care*. 1997;(suppl 3):S21–S32.

45. Fetterolf D, West R. The business case for quality: Combining medical literature research with health plan data to establish value for non-clinical managers. *American Journal of Medical Quality*. March/April 2004;19(2):48–55.

46. Academy of Healthcare Management. Health Plan Finance and Risk Management. Atlanta, GA: Academy for Healthcare Management. 1999.

Chapter 5

MEDICAL INFORMATICS AND INFORMATION SYSTEMS:

THE INFORMATION INFRASTRUCTURE NEEDED TO SUPPORT QUALITY MEASUREMENT AND IMPROVEMENT

Louis H. Diamond, MB, ChB

Introduction

This chapter is focused on the information infrastructure needed to support quality measurement. Health care delivery is essentially an information exchange between the patient and health care professional, and among health care professionals. The components of such an information infrastructure include the medical record, elements of the medical record (such as a personal health record and continuity of care records), point-of-care decision-support tools, and performance measurement systems. All these components support both individual patient management as well as the management of patient populations. Connectivity between patients and members of the health care delivery team and between team members is an essential component of the needed information infrastructure.

An IOM Report (1990) on Medicare and Quality defines health care quality as "the degree to which health services for individuals and populations increase the likelihood of desired health outcomes and are consistent with current professional knowledge." Events that adversely affect health care quality fall into three categories: underuse, overuse, and misuse of care.[1-3] Overuse occurs when the care provided is unnecessary, may put patient safety at risk, and results in the unneeded delivery of costly services. Underuse is the failure to provide people with needed care, including preventive services. Misuse, which includes medical errors, a process event, adverse events, an outcome, is the inappropriate execution of a planned event.

⬤ Development of an Information Infrastructure: Historical Background

The United States lacks a robust comprehensive measurement set to assess health care quality. Instead, a variety of mechanisms measures disparate aspects of health care quality. Leaders in the public and private sectors are demanding national goals for quality improvement as well as standardized measures for tracking these improvements at the national level and across facility types. The National Quality Forum has begun the process of adopting such a quality measurement set.

Legislation covering a broad spectrum of health care quality issues has been enacted in many states. At the federal level, various legislative initiatives have been introduced, and the executive branch has moved swiftly to coordinate a wide range of projects across federal agencies.

In recent years, the health care industry, major employers, and health care professionals have tried to measure the quality of health care. In 1997, the Joint Commission on Accreditation of Healthcare Organizations (JCAHO), which provides accreditation services for almost 19,000 health care organizations, launched the ORYX initiative as part of its accreditation process.[4] In 2003–4, JCAHO has moved to incorporate an expanded quality measurement into the accreditation process. Since 1997, the National Committee for Quality Assurance (NCQA) has compared the performance of health care plans on selected quality measures; NCQA currently assesses 237 health care plans nationwide.[5] The National Quality Forum (NQF), a not-for-profit membership organization created in 1999 to develop a national strategy for health care quality measurement and reporting, has designed a framework for selecting performance measures.[6] As part of its mission, the NQF is evaluating and endorsing measurement sets for hospitals and nursing homes, has endorsed a nursing sensitive quality measurement set, and, in 2004, has commenced efforts to measure physician performance for a group of high-priority diseases, such as diabetes, hypertension, hyperlipidemia, and certain types of cancer.

The Leapfrog Group, formed in 2000, consists of Fortune 500 companies and other large health care consumer advocacy groups that are committed to improving safety in health care through purchasing decisions that reward providers who promote quality improvement efforts.[7] The effort by the Leapfrog Group is an attempt to bridge the gap in quality performance and to enhance the ability of purchasers (employers) and patients to become more prudent buyers. They have initially identified three sets of services that they believe will substantially enhance quality of service and reduce costs. These "leaps," as they are called, are computerized physician order entry, ICU coverage by intensivists, and evidence-based referral to hospitals that perform these services above a stated threshold. In 2004, additional "leaps" have been added, now with a focus on the physicians' office setting. By requiring these services to be in place and releasing compliance information to their employees, the Leapfrog Group hopes to help facilitate change.

In 1999, the Institute of Medicine (IOM) issued a report entitled *To Err Is Human: Building a Safer Health System*. Based on an extrapolation of data supplied by the Harvard Medical Practice Study and other sources, the report claimed that 44,000 to 98,000 Americans might die annually as a result of medical errors.[8] The report captured the attention of the public and of policymakers at federal and state levels. It drew national interest to the quality of health care, how it is measured, and how it can be improved.

In *To Err Is Human: Building a Safer Health System* (Institute of Medicine, 1999a), the dimensions of quality are described as safety; practice consistent with current, evidence-based medical knowledge; and customization that accounts for the personal preference of the patient.

Figure 5–1	A Model of the Influence of External Drives on Quality

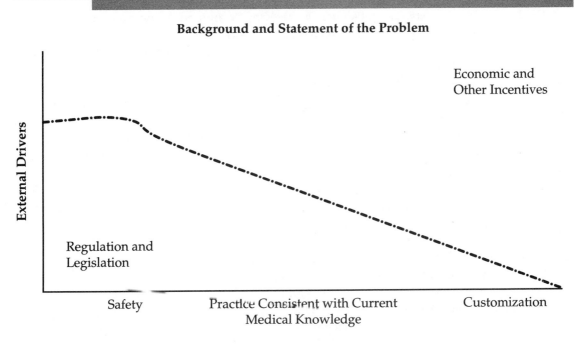

Background and Statement of the Problem

Economic and
Other Incentives

External Drivers

Regulation and
Legislation

Safety   Practice Consistent with Current   Customization
                        Medical Knowledge

Domains of Quality

Source: Kohn LT, et al. *To Err is Human: Building a Safer Health System.* IOM. 1999.

This construct needs to be interpreted with regard to overuse, underuse, and misuse. External drivers for improving the dimensions of quality range from regulation and legislation to economic market forces (see Figure 5–1). Within this paradigm, safety becomes the de facto "floor" of quality—a necessary, but not a sufficient, requirement. Regulation and legislation are predominantly designed to influence safety, whereas economic and other incentives influence evidence-based care and customization.

This IOM report followed an earlier 1998 report by the President's Advisory Commission on Consumer Protection and Quality in the Health Care Industry, entitled *Quality First: Better Health Care for All Americans.* This report identified quality as a major problem, and called for a national commitment to improving the quality of health care. Released one year later by the IOM, *To Err Is Human: Building a Safer Health System* recommended establishing nationwide, mandatory, or voluntary reporting systems; creating a national patient safety center to set goals; tracking progress and developing a national research agenda; making safety a primary concern to consumers, professionals, and accreditation groups; and developing a culture of safety among health care organizations.[8]

In 2001, the IOM produced two additional quality-related reports: *Envisioning the National Health Care Quality Report*[9] and *Crossing the Quality Chasm: A New Health Care System for the 21st Century.*[10] The *Chasm* report argued that a chasm exists between the quality of care that *is* provided and the quality that *could* be provided. It called for organizing evidence-based care processes and developing the necessary information infrastructure to support the provision and ongoing measurement of quality care. This report called for a renewed commitment to patient-centeredness, to evidence-based medicine, and to a system-oriented team approach to the delivery of health care.

The *Envisioning the National Health Care Quality Report* proposed "a context of accountability" for the entire health care system. It pictured a quality report composed of public and private data source elements. Specifically, the quality report is meant to propose recommendations for designing and implementing a "balanced scorecard" or "dashboard" of quality indicators and measures. The annual report is expected to enhance the awareness of quality, to define the context of accountability for improvement, to monitor the possible effects of policy decisions and initiatives on quality, and to assess the progress in attaining national health care goals.

These IOM reports possessed several common themes. Each called for expanding quality measurement and reporting and suggesting that implementation of these quality measurement systems would require creating an information infrastructure, using evidence-based medicine, and enhancing patient participation. This agenda is anticipated to require collaborative leadership from the public and private sectors, as well as substantial investment in education and training for health care professionals.

Technology can enhance health care quality and quality measurement in various ways. It increases accuracy and timeliness, enables up-to-date evidence and decision support systems to be used at the point of patient care, improves coordination among clinicians and between patients and clinicians, and enhances the capacity to collect and report information on performance.[10] Furthermore, technology can determine the extent to which health plans can capture relevant data for quality measures and the degree to which policymakers are able to measure improvement in health care over time.

Evidence-based medicine, defined as "the integration of best research evidence with clinical expertise and patient values," implies the use of clinically relevant research, systematic reviews of multiple primary investigations (including meta-analyses), or evidence-based practice guidelines.[11] Evidence-based medicine can lead to effective delivery of health care services based on scientific knowledge and to avoidance of the pitfalls of misuse, overuse, or underuse.[10]

An improved information infrastructure can help evidence-based medicine be applied clinically by allowing clinicians to access, either in the clinician's office or at the patient's bedside, patient health information and electronic medical literature about best practices and population-based data. In addition, evidence-based "alert systems" can aid decisionmaking by members of the professional team and by the patient. Finally, technology offers the capacity to increase the speed with which new information about clinical practices is generated and disseminated to practitioners, especially regarding the provisions of performance information, a necessary but insufficient requirement to facilitate provider behavioral change and system re-engineering.

Leading the health care system through such fundamental systemic and technological change requires leadership by the public and private sectors. The identification, dissemination, and application of evidence-based practice—the use of evidence-based quality measures assisted by information technology—will require extensive public and private collaboration.[10]

Improvements in technology will require considerable, and continual, educational efforts to ensure that health professionals develop new skills and keep abreast of new developments. The health care workforce must be prepared to better serve patients in a world of expanding knowledge and rapid change. This goal may demand that licensure and certification reflect these new necessary professional skills.[10] Investments in the health services research capacity will also be necessary to ensure that the rich data generated by information technology are analyzed and used.

The Purpose and Philosophy of an Information Infrastructure

Developing an expanded information infrastructure to improve health care quality has two overarching purposes: (1) to assist clinicians in treating and coordinating the care of an individual patient at the point of care, and (2) to facilitate individual patient management in concert with the health care needs of a given population. The former, essentially the operational system (i.e., a component of the computerized medical record), will not be addressed in this chapter; however, the latter will be dealt with. The component needed for performance measurement and to support disease management and related activities will be described as "Populations," which is used in broad terms, and covers populations as multiple levels (e.g., an individual physician's patient population, or a health plan's populations). To fulfill the first purpose, a computerized (electronic) medical record (EMR) that contains digital information is envisaged, including diagnostic data such as physical exams, patient medical history, laboratory and radiograph results, medication information, presence of other diseases or co-morbidities, and a description of treatment plans. In addition, clinicians can have electronic access to the health literature and analysis of population-level data when making diagnoses and deciding among therapeutic approaches.[10] Furthermore, clinical decision support systems (CDSS) can integrate patient-specific information with a computerized knowledge base to assist a clinical assessment or decisionmaking. Such systems may also generate reminders and have been shown to improve adherence with clinical practice guidelines.[12]

Additional patient-specific, real-time, point-of-care clinical decision support instruments that go beyond reminders are also being researched. These efforts are being undertaken because, at the point of care, physicians need to understand their patients' probable clinical outcome trajectory, and the combinations of clinical decisions that will achieve that patient's optimal short-term and long-term clinical outcomes. This information could enable clinicians to consider "mid-course corrections" (alternative decisions) that take into account changes in the patient's presentation and that could allow them to model the potential effects of different clinical decisions on the patient's clinical course changes.

The second purpose of the information infrastructure, facilitating individual patient management in concert with the health care needs of a given population, is the primary focus of this chapter. By aggregating patient-level data, information systems generate population-level data that can be analyzed to assess the health care performance of systems and of health care professionals, as well as to enable research on health care processes and outcomes. Most existing information systems are not designed for these multiplicative purposes.[3] Significant investment is needed in population-level health information systems to advance evidence-based health care, support continued research and innovation, and compare performance of health plans, hospitals, facilities, and practitioners.

Centralizing clinical-case, patient-level databases can provide insights into clinical practice. Population-level analyses allow clinicians to compare their actual performance with a stated goal. This process enables clinicians to compare their ideal clinical behavior with their current practice patterns, thus catalyzing an objective, data-driven basis for change management. These analyses enable cross-institutional and cross-regional comparison of health care quality and practitioner performance. In addition, linking population assessment with real-time decision support increases clinical decision support-system value by leveraging the power of the analysis of large population-based clinical information.

⬤ Components of an Information Infrastructure for Quality Management

An information infrastructure that is designed to advance quality management must meet public and private sector needs. Therefore, information infrastructure should allow private and public groups to track progress against established national goals, and it should also allow all groups to meet internal management needs and provide for a national public reporting system. A key component is a multidimensional performance measurement set.

A conceptual framework, described by the Strategic Framework Board of the National Quality Forum (NQF) and now endorsed by the NQF's full Board of Directors, outlines two measurement pathways as components of an information infrastructure for supporting quality management. One pathway supports quality improvement, whereas the other supports accountability and choice (see Figure 5–2).

The main components of the information infrastructure are data sources; data definitions; coding (or classification) systems; data transmission; data storage, management, and analysis; quality measurement; and reporting techniques. These components are described in subsequent subsections.

Data Sources

The first steps to consider when improving the health information infrastructure are defining the measurement needs, identifying the data sources and those available in existing systems, and then identifying gaps. Approached from a national perspective, the Agency for Healthcare Research and Quality (AHRQ) has been commissioned by the U.S. Congress to produce an annual report that captures the status of quality in the delivery of health care. In turn, AHRQ commissioned the Institute of Medicine to produce a conceptual framework for such a report, to articulate the components of health care quality to be measured, and to identify potential data sources. The Institute of Medicine identified the four components of health care quality to be safety, effectiveness, patient-centeredness, and timeliness.

In *Envisioning the National Health Care Quality Report*, the Institute of Medicine outlined existing public and private data sources that have the potential to address one or more of these four components of quality. Criteria for inclusion as a data source included credibility and validity, national scope (with the potential to provide state-level detail), availability and consistency over time, timeliness, the potential for subgroup and condition-specific analysis, and public accessibility.[9] The report also suggests that long- and short-term perspectives are required in planning for data collection and coordination for health care quality assessment at the national level, and several recommendations are made.[9] Over the next decade, data must be gathered from a collection of existing sources. Patient surveys should be used to collect data on patient-centeredness and timeliness, and claims data should capture information on safety and effectiveness. "Gaps" should be spanned using information from targeted medical record abstraction. In the longer term, a new health information infrastructure based on existing and new data sources, including electronic clinical data systems, new population surveys, and specialized data systems, will be required to meet national health care quality measurement goals.

Data are potentially available from a wide variety of sources, including claims data; hard-copy information, such as medical records; and formal systems that provide payment information, such as claims and survey data. Some of these data are available to organizations electronically through internal systems.

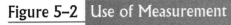

Figure 5-2   Use of Measurement

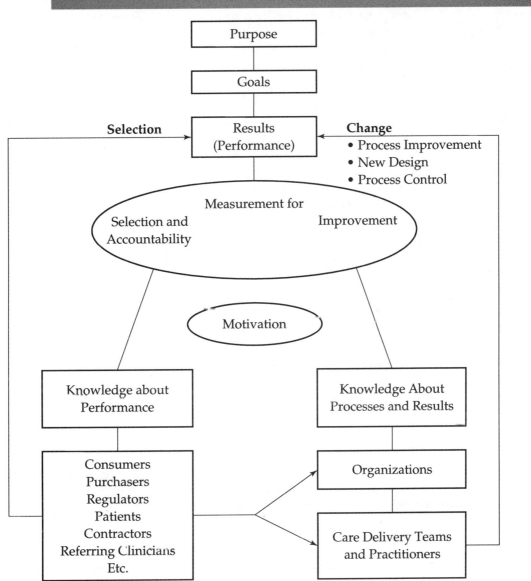

Source: Adapted from: Berwick, DM. The Connections Between Measurement and Improvement. NQF Board Mtg. 11/29/00.

Data Definitions

The quality of data in an information infrastructure depends on the degree to which the data captures—with completeness, detail, and accuracy—the concepts of interest. Sound communication of health care information requires a common understanding of terms. In health care information systems, "terminology" refers to health care terms and their definitions that are communicated numerically through combinations of coded data elements. A "data set" refers to a commonly agreed upon collection of data elements that are used for defining a clinical domain. Terms associated with this process include "terminology," "classification," and "nomenclature" and are largely used interchangeably. Technically, the more precise "nomenclatures" are aggregated to form "classifications," and the continuum from one to the other is referred to collectively as "terminology."[13]

Presently, over 150 clinically related classification systems, nomenclatures, dictionaries, terminologies, vocabulary lists, and code sets are used in the United States.[13] Each classification system was designed to meet a specific need, such as physician reimbursement. Each system differs in the extent to which it is general or disease- or domain-specific. Furthermore, not only the content but also the structure of the classification system varies. One system may use hierarchical codes associated with terms, whereas another may impart definitions related to terms. In creating a health care information infrastructure, a mechanism for combining these various systems is desirable.[13]

Building the future information infrastructure will require developing a system of measures that are universally standardized and understood, much as the metric system offers a standardized system for measurements. Standard terminology enables data capture to proceed in a structured manner, thereby facilitating the collection of information and enhancing the ability to perform data analyses.[14] Efficient health care delivery depends on accurate and detailed clinical information. The more detailed, reliable, and comparable the data, the more valuable is its contribution to best practices, decision support tools, and other mechanisms designed to enhance the quality of health care.

In addition to standardized classification systems, terminologies and coding systems must be expanded. Present coding schemes are not sufficiently comprehensive to capture the level of clinical precision desirable for quality measurement purposes.[15] In many instances, coding schemes do not capture all clinical services. Progress in expanding the terminology of some areas of health care is being made. For example, major efforts are underway to incorporate terminology that captures nursing diagnoses and interventions.[16] Such developments are important for facilitating the reimbursement of nursing services and for documenting the contribution of nursing services to patient care outcomes.

Coding Classification Systems

An essential building block for constructing and implementing a health information infrastructure is the adoption of classification systems and standards for the data elements, including data transmission, storage, and analysis; and use of the data. What follows is an outline of some of these dimensions.

1. *International Classification of Diseases (ICD)*. The health care system in the United States uses the International Classification of Diseases, Version 9, and Clinical Modification for Use in the United States (ICD-9-CM) as its official system of assigning codes to diagnoses and procedures that apply to hospital use. The classification system is used for provider reimbursement, quality review, and benchmarking measurements. Based on the World Health Organization's classification system, the Tenth Revision of the International Classification of Diseases (ICD-10) is used to code and classify mortality data from death certificates. In the United States, the National Center for Health Statistics (NCHS) and the Center for Medicare and Medicaid Services (CMS) manage the system and modify it to meet the particular needs of the nation's evolving health care system.[17] Current efforts are underway to complete a Clinical Modification of the ICD-10 diagnoses (ICD-10-CM). Additionally, CMS has already completed the development of an ICD-10 companion Procedural Classification System (ICD-10-PCS). This classification system has the adaptability and flexibility to

accommodate new technologies more quickly than has been the case with ICD-9-CM procedural classification updates.

2. *Current Procedural Terminology (CPT)*. A system used for classifying clinical procedures and services performed by physicians is the Current Procedural Terminology, Fourth Edition (CPT-4). The system is developed under the auspices of the American Medical Association (AMA) and is used by accreditation organizations; by payers for administrative, financial, and analytical purposes; and by researchers for outcomes studies, public health initiatives, and health services research. Efforts are underway to develop the next generation of CPT (CPT-5). The new system is designed to respond to the challenges of the Health Insurance Portability and Accountability Act of 1996 (HIPAA) and supports electronic interfaces. Specifically, CPT-5 is designed to communicate easily with demographic information systems, electronic health records, and analytical databases of varying levels of detail. It is anticipated that CPT-5 will be the standard for reporting physician's services under HIPAA regulations.

3. *Systematized Nomenclature of Medicine (SNOMED)*. Used in more than 40 countries, the Systematized Nomenclature of Medicine (SNOMED) represents a broad array of health care concepts.[16] SNOMED was created for indexing the entire medical record, including signs and symptoms, diagnoses, and procedures. It is being adopted worldwide as the standard for indexing medical records information. SNOMED may be used for disease management, health services research, outcomes research, and quality improvement analyses. It is promoted as a system through which detailed clinical information can be shared across specialties, sites of care, and various information system platforms.

4. *Unified Medical Language System (UMLS)*. Developed by the National Library of Medicine, the Unified Medical Language System provides an electronic link between clinical vocabularies and medical literature from disparate sources.[13] The goal is to develop a means whereby a wide variety of application programs can overcome retrieval problems caused by differences in terminology and the scattering of relevant information across many databases. For example, UMLS eases the linkage between computer-based patient records, bibliographic databases, factual databases, and expert systems. The National Library of Medicine distributes annual editions, free-of-charge under a license agreement, and encourages feedback, which promotes expansion of the database. "The Metathesaurus" provides a uniform, integrated distribution format from more than 60 biomedical vocabularies and classifications, and links many different names for the same concepts. "The Lexicon" contains syntactic information for many terms, component words, and English words (including verbs) that do not appear in the Metathesaurus. "The Semantic Network" contains information about the types or categories to which all Metathesaurus concepts have been assigned (e.g., "Disease or Syndrome," "Virus") and the permissible relationships among these types (e.g., "Virus" causes "Disease or Syndrome").[18]

5. *Logical Observation Identifiers, Names, and Codes (LOINC)*. The development of a system known as Logical Observation Identifiers, Names, and Codes (LOINC) originally focused on a public use set of codes and names for electronic reporting of laboratory test results.[16] It has been expanded to encompass a database of names, synonyms, and codes, and it can also capture clinical measurements, such as EKG data.[19] LOINC content is continually expanding to include more direct patient measurements and clinical observations.[16] LOINC data are available from the Regenstrief HL7

website.[20] An extensive review of these needed standards is described in a recent IOM report entitled, "Developing a Safer Healthcare System."[21]

Data Transmission

Data transmission is a critical component of the information infrastructure. As with terminology and coding, standardization is needed to improve efficiency in the electronic transmission of data. Electronic health care data transmission issues include the need for a transmission mechanism, format and content standards, a unique identifier to ensure that records are appropriately assigned to the correct individual, assurance of data confidentiality, and mechanisms to ensure data security. These issues have received widespread attention, as epitomized in the Health Insurance Portability and Accountability Act of 1996 (HIPAA), which mandates:

1. Standards for electronic data interchange transactions
2. Standards for code sets
3. The use of unique patient identifiers
4. Policies and procedures to assure security and privacy.[22]

Data that are stored in different formats need to be mapped and translated. In the absence of standardization, translations often must be performed manually. Such translations are costly, and each data transaction comes with the potential for error. The standardization of data formats and elements can eliminate this cumbersome step. At present, many health care organizations rely on Health Level Seven (HL-7) for this standardization function. HL-7 is "a not-for-profit, ANSI-accredited standards development organization whose mission is to provide standards for the exchange, management, and integration of medical data that support clinical patient care and the management, delivery, and evaluation of health care services."[16] HL-7 supports an application protocol for the electronic exchange of clinical and associated administrative data.[19] The application communicates orders, referrals, diagnostic results, and visit notes across health care entities. HL-7 may be thought of as a standard for the data structure for records that are sent between individual systems, the content and terminologies of which are constantly being revised and expanded to meet various health informatics needs.[19]

A controversial and important issue in health care data transmission is the use of a unique patient identifier. The unique identifier can enable an individual's lifetime experience with the health care system to be accessed electronically. The Computer-Based Patient Record Institute claims that the present lack of a unique patient identifier frequently leads to health care data not being correctly matched to the appropriate patient.[13] The development of a unique health care identifier was included in the 1996 HIPAA legislation, because without it the potential of electronic health care data systems was expected to remain largely untapped. However, HIPAA privacy concerns have caused the issue of a unique patient identifier to be placed on hold indefinitely.

The privacy concerns surrounding the use of a unique patient identifier are substantial. For example, there are concerns that if social security numbers are used, a linkage to non–health care data could occur. To address these concerns, a variety of non-numeric approaches to a unique identifier, including DNA prints and thumbprints, have been proposed.[13] However, it appears that even the transmission of this information would require translation to a numeric base.

To ensure that privacy and security concerns are addressed, applying a universal unique health care identifier system would require strict enforcement of rules governing the linking of data and the prevention of unauthorized access to confidential data. Mechanisms, such as encryption and secure networks, would need to ensure data security. Furthermore, national consideration would have to be given to the organization that is charged with overseeing the implementation and use of a unique identifier. For example, if the social security number was used, the Social Security Administration might provide the necessary oversight.

Under the 1996 HIPAA privacy and confidentiality rules, health care information is considered confidential and can only be shared for the purposes of treatment, payment, and health care organization operation without the explicit permission of the patient. However, it is recognized that information about treatment outcomes, disease trends, and risk factors is derived from studies that use personally identifiable data. Therefore, for research purposes (among academic institutions, federal and state government agencies, pharmaceutical manufacturers, and other entities), individually identifiable data may be used if the research design is approved by the necessary institutional research review boards and confirmed to safeguard patient safety.

HIPAA regulations require that "covered entities" implement policies and procedures on the use of individually identifiable data and its confidentiality and security. "Covered entities" include only those providers and payers who transmit standard administrative transactions to each other. HIPAA regulations also mandate that "covered entities" have guidelines for:

1. The administration of information security systems
2. Education programs on confidentiality and security
3. Confidentiality agreements
4. Access control
5. Authorizations for release of information
6. Authentication mechanisms
7. Functional requirements for maintaining data integrity
8. Log-on procedures
9. Audit trails
10. Disaster prevention and recovery
11. Data storage and transmission

Guidelines for data storage and transmission are needed because evidence-based clinical practice guidelines and derived clinical performance measures are critical for successful disease management.

Data Storage and Analysis

Once data are collected and transmitted, they must be stored. Once stored, they must be accessible and easy to analyze so that they can be reported.

Web interfaces for clinical systems exist, and the variety of Web applications is likely to expand rapidly.[23, 24] This use of the Web for data storage and analysis raises a number of issues, including whether the general population has access to the Internet. The future patient-centered health care environment is envisioned as a place where patients will have electronic access to information on quality indicators and to their own medical records. Electronic communication between health care professionals and patients is also expected to be widely used.[25, 26]

Data Storage.

How data are stored has important implications for their use. The storage method should allow providers, patients, managers, and others to access the data in a format that meets their particular needs. The separate functions of three common data storage systems—operational data stores, data

Table 5-1	Data Characteristics

Operational Data	Decision Support Data
➡ Primitive	➡ Derived
➡ Detailed (atomic)	➡ Summarized
➡ Current	➡ Historical value over time
➡ Transaction/process oriented	➡ Analysis or subject oriented
➡ Volatile (frequent updates)	➡ Non-volatile (infrequent updates)
➡ One record at a time	➡ Time-variant snapshots, multiple records
➡ Repetitive	➡ Heuristic
➡ Performance optimized	➡ Performance relaxed
➡ Presentation (output) difficult	➡ Presentation optimized
➡ No redundancy (normalized)	➡ Redundancy acceptable (denormalized)
➡ Serves "production" function	➡ Serves managerial function
➡ High accessibility	➡ Modest accessibility
➡ Static structure, variable contents	➡ Flexible structure

Source: Bush D. Why is data warehousing failing us? *Managed Healthcare News.* 2000;16(6).

warehouses, and data marts—must be recognized. Operational data stores drive clinical decision support systems (CDSS), which are clinical consultation systems that use population statistics combined with expert knowledge to offer real-time information to clinicians. The focus of these systems is individual patient management, and patient-specific information is included in the analysis. Such systems are useful in day-to-day operational decisions.[27]

Data warehouses differ fundamentally from operational data stores; data warehouses are designed for strategic decision support rather than for operational decision support.[27]

Often referred to as "health care archaeology," data warehouses generally store information from a three- to five-year period and are used to evaluate clinical and financial performance in groups of patients *after* care has been given. A data warehouse is a centralized repository of a single copy of corporate integrated data that comes from a variety of sources.[28, 29] It serves the needs of the entire organization and typically includes data from sources such as claims, providers, pharmacies, laboratories, and materials management. The data warehouse has analytic and querying functions and can specifically analyze clinical and financial information for purposes of utilization review, component cost evaluation, and clinician performance evaluation.[27]

The data warehouse and the operational data store have distinct functions and are designed differently (see Table 5–1). The operational data store offers real-time data, is process-oriented, provides data in textual output, and serves a distinctly operational function. In contrast, the data warehouse maintains historical data summarized in analytical aggregates, and its analytical paths are loosely structured to facilitate varied investigations. The data warehouse offers graphical presentations of information, and serves a managerial function.[27]

Although the data warehouse holds important information for population analysis, the large volume of data that it contains often makes it cumbersome. The data warehouse has a primary purpose of storing cleansed and constructing data marts to support specific purposes. Data marts are department-oriented, smaller in scope, less expensive to manage, and less time-consuming to construct. They are built for a specific analytical purpose and serve a small group of analysts. A data mart offers improved accessibility to the data, and few maintenance issues for the database ad-

Figure 5–3   Data Repositories: High-Level Architecture

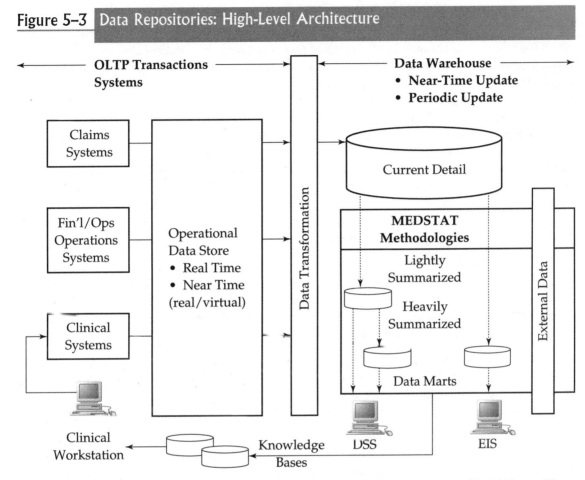

Source: Adapted from RE Gilbreath, Heath care data repositories: Components and a model. *Healthc Inf Manage.* Winter 1995;9(1):63–73.

ministrator.[29] Once data have been aggregated in a data mart, they are easier to manipulate for analysis (see Figure 5–3).

Data Analysis.

Collecting and maintaining health care information and having an information infrastructure are prerequisite investments for analytic support of quality measurement and management. Because no two patients are identical, analysis of health care data presents special challenges to investigators who wish to study processes of care or medical outcomes.

When patients are grouped for statistical or comparative studies, risk adjustment methodologies are used to remove the effect of (i.e., to control for) patient differences. Risk adjustment is used for many purposes. Physicians and hospitals apply risk adjustment in quality management by grouping patients with similar prognoses when conducting outcomes studies. Providers also use risk adjustment in analyzing prospective payment and evaluating costs. Health plans, public payers, and employers use risk adjustment techniques in evaluating hospital and physician performance and in setting prospective payment rates.

A common theme in risk adjustment is the notion of making "apples-to-apples" comparisons by accounting for pertinent patient and environmental characteristics before making inferences about the effectiveness or quality of care based on patient outcomes. Patient characteristics that are typically controlled for include age, sex, race, diagnoses, severity of illness, and physical functioning. Outcomes frequently include mortality, chronic disease and morbidity, complications of care, the costs of care, and patient satisfaction.

Interest in risk adjustment techniques has grown. Today, many well-known and respected methodologies can be integrated in a data warehouse for use in outcomes studies, provider profiling analyses, payment development, and forecasting. Among the better-known risk-adjustment methodologies are Diagnosis-Related Groups, All Patient Refined Diagnosis-Related Groups, Disease Staging, Episodes, Episodic Treatment Groups, Episode Groupers, Resource Use Methods, Ambulatory Clinical Conditions, and Diagnostic Cost Groups. These risk-adjustment and severity-of-illness methods have been designed to quantify risk for hospitalized patients. They are used in hospital payment calculations and to monitor clinical efficiency and hospital costs.

1. *Diagnosis-Related Groups (DRGs)*. In DRGs, patients are categorized into one of 498 DRGs by diagnosis, major surgical procedure, age, sex, and the presence of a complication or co-morbidity. Diagnosis-related groups, which are homogeneous groupings with respect to hospital charges and length of stay, are best known for their use in Medicare hospital payments, but they are also used for comparative hospital cost and efficiency studies.

2. *All Patient Refined Diagnosis-Related Groups (APR-DRGs)*. This methodology uses the DRG case-mix schema with diagnosis-based severity levels to account for a patient's level of illness. Although the underlying DRG structure is resource-based, clinical judgment and empirical testing are used in designing and validating the severity levels.

3. *Disease Staging*. Disease staging consists of two risk adjustment methodologies. The first is predicated on the progression of disease and involves documenting increasing levels of severity, known as disease stages. More than 600 diseases are distinguished, and patients may fall into more than one disease category based on the number of diagnoses recorded on a hospital claim. The Disease Staging Charge, Length of Stay, and Mortality scales form the basis of the second risk-adjustment technique. The scales are patient-level forecasts of expected resource use and in-hospital mortality.

4. *Episodes*. The unit of analysis for episode risk-adjustment techniques is a clinically defined course of illness. In-patient and out-patient claims and encounters are associated with an episode. An episode ends after a period during which no claims are encountered and the patient is assumed to have recovered from an acute illness or condition. Chronic episodes typically are open-ended and accumulate claims for the duration of the study period.

5. *Episodic Treatment Groups (ETGs)*. The methodology of ETGs uses homogeneous treatment episodes that categorize patients by disease condition and medical or surgical intervention. Cost weights profile the efficiency of treatment of patients by physicians.

6. *MEDSTAT Episode Grouper (MEG)*. In the MEG methodology, episodes are constructed around the disease or medical condition of a patient, regardless of treatment. Each episode is constructed from Disease Staging by disease categories and severity. The method enables users to compare and contrast the timing and appropriateness of medical interventions.

7. *Resource Use Methods.* Diagnosis-based risk adjustment methods calculate risk-adjusted payments to physicians and hospitals. These resource-use methods are employed in disease management and provider profiling studies.

8. *Ambulatory Clinical Groupings (ACGs).* The methodology of ACGs is constructed by using the diagnoses and patient demographics found on in-patient and out-patient claims. Patients are categorized into a single ACG based on demographic information and their diagnoses over the study period. In a few cases, an ACG is related to specific medical conditions. However, most of the groups are broad (e.g., "Chronic Medical," "Unstable").

9. *Diagnostic Cost Groups (DCGs).* The original purpose of the DCG risk-adjustment methodology was to design a method for administering prospective ambulatory care payments to physicians. Initially, diagnoses from in-patient and out-patient claims are grouped into 543 diagnostic groups. These groups are further collapsed into 118 Hierarchical Condition Categories (HCCs). Based on a patient's HCC, statistical forecasts reflect the incremental cost of each condition. Populations may be stratified by sociodemographic attributes (age, sex, insurance status, and various socioeconomic attributes), as well as by measures of health status. This case-mix adjustment methodology predicts a population's past or future health care utilization and costs. Various grouping applications, such as Adjusted Clinical Groups (ACGs), Diagnostic Cost Groups (DCGs), and Disease Staging applications may be used. These types of categorizations and analyses are important for quality improvement investigations because they "level the playing field" by taking into account the level of illness of the patient under care.

Various types of adjustment approaches are in common use. ACGs use claims and encounter information to group individuals who are likely to have similar resource requirements, on the theory that level of health is associated with level of health care resource use. ACGs use ICD-9 diagnosis codes and demographic information to assign individuals to one of 83 mutually exclusive categories that are found to have similar resource requirements. Similarly, DCGs require ICD-9 diagnosis data from claims and encounter data, where groupings are based on expenditures of samples of Medicare recipients. Disease staging is a way of adjusting for variation in patient clinical severity, which is based on the concept that diseases naturally progress through stages. The assumption is that these stages can be measured independently of the services provided.

Quality Measurement

A balanced set of cost, use, and quality measures is needed to support a robust effort to assess health care value. The Strategic Framework Board of the National Quality Forum has provided a road map for both national and local quality measurement and reporting initiatives.[6] Defining the goals of a measurement system is an essential first step. The National Quality Forum describes two pathways, one to support accountability and be used by patients in selecting a physician, and the second to support internal quality improvement efforts. These two pathways are connected and need to be deployed in parallel. Further criteria for selecting quality measures are the cost and incidence of the disease, and the aspects of care being assessed. Conditions of high cost and high frequency are important, as is the evidence base for the dimension of quality being measured.

Quality measurement is limited by the data sources that support the measures. The most useful quality measures contain a well described, evidentiary linkage between process and outcome. Without such a linkage, neither a process nor an outcome is useful as a quality performance measure. The aspect of care being measured must be controllable by the group being assessed, with the expectation that changes can improve quality. A spectrum of the representation aspects of data sources, the process-outcome linkage, and accountability is given in Figure 5–4.

Each vector in Figure 5–4 illustrates the complexity of clinical performance measures (CPMs) and quality measures (QMs). The term "quality measure" is used to capture the measurement of quality, which is based on an accepted definition of quality and a quality indicator, or an indirect measurement of quality. The term "performance measurement" is used when the quality measurement documents the actual performance of a provider, hospital, or physician, when the quality dimension being measured is under the direct control of the provider. In contrast, in a quality measure, attribution of responsibility might be unclear.

The word "spectrum" in Figure 5–4 connotes a fluidity of movement from left to right. The figure is anchored on the left by "use" measures and on the right by the most robust "quality" measures. The progression of measures from left to right is illustrated with diabetes. Throughout the following discussion, a measure on the far left of the spectrum is compared with one on the far right to point out the distinctions between the extremes. Evidence-based medicine (EBM) finds an application in the development of CPMs. Evidence gleaned from the medical literature is synthesized into a clinical practice guideline (CPG), an authoritative statement used as a guide in decision-making by both members of the health care delivery team and the patient. The codification of the evidence in the CPGs is the foundation for developing CPMs. For example, the CPGs of the American Diabetes Association recommend yearly examinations by an eye specialist for patients with diabetes. Such exams can find retinal disease early and allow for timely intervention to prevent or delay loss of vision. As a measure moves from the left to the right in the figure, better and clearer

Figure 5–4   Use/Quality Measures Spectrum

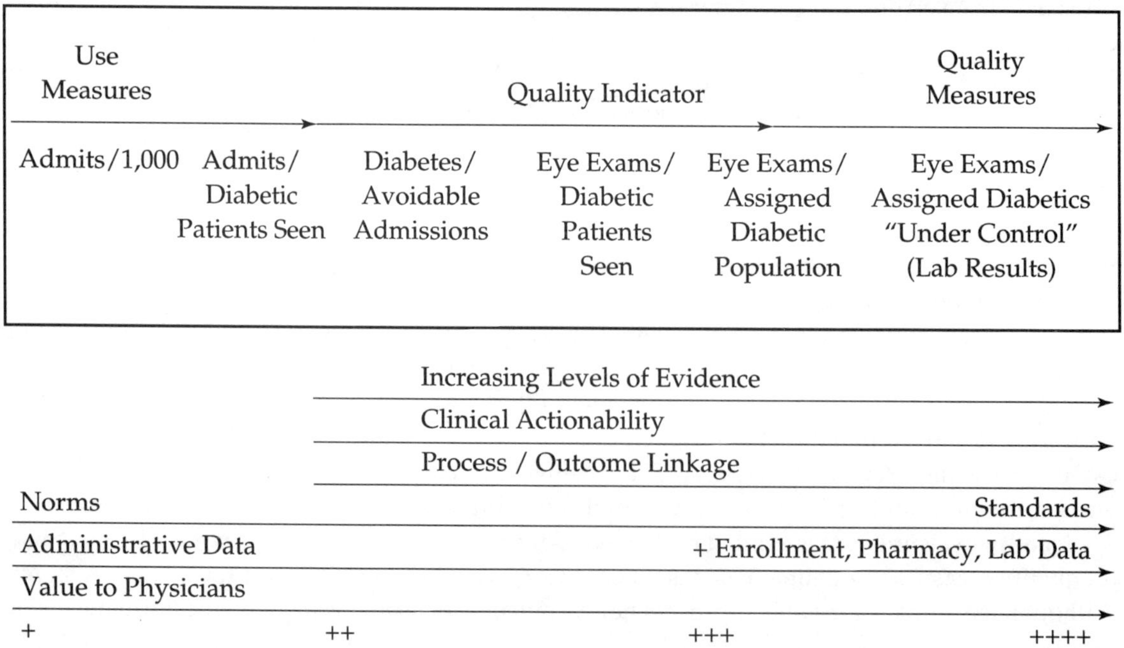

Use Measures			Quality Indicator		Quality Measures
Admits/1,000	Admits/ Diabetic Patients Seen	Diabetes/ Avoidable Admissions	Eye Exams/ Diabetic Patients Seen	Eye Exams/ Assigned Diabetic Population	Eye Exams/ Assigned Diabetics "Under Control" (Lab Results)

Increasing Levels of Evidence →

Clinical Actionability →

Process / Outcome Linkage →

Norms	Standards →
Administrative Data	+ Enrollment, Pharmacy, Lab Data →
Value to Physicians	→

| + | ++ | +++ | ++++ |

evidence is required to support it. In contrast, a "use" measure, such as admissions per 1,000 patients, has no evidence to support it. Although there may be general agreement that admissions to U.S. hospitals are "too high," it is unclear what the admission rate should be. In addition, this measure examines all admissions for 1,000 patients of any age, sex, or ethnicity and with any diagnosis.

"Actionability" refers to the clarity of what should be done and who should do it. As a measure moves from the left to right in the figure, what needs to be done and by whom becomes clearer. For example, if the measure looks at yearly eye examinations for patients with diabetes, the action is to conduct eye examinations for patients with diabetes sometime during a one-year period; in addition, actionability implies a component of responsibility. In this example, the primary care physician is the one who orders the examination, the eye care specialist is the one who performs the examination, and the patient with diabetes is the one who receives the examination. With the admissions per 1,000 measure, it is unclear what action should be taken to affect this rate, who should take the action, and which patients should be involved in the action.

A good clinical performance measure requires a strong link between process (what is done to, for, or by the patient) and outcome (the result of applying the process). Such links are found in the systematic reviews and meta-analyses that form the basis of evidence-based medicine. In the diabetes example, an evidence-based link exists between yearly eye examinations for patients with diabetes (process) and the delay or minimizing of eye complications (outcome). Therefore, measuring the rate of yearly eye examinations for patients with diabetes and increasing this rate, if necessary, could result in "better" ocular functioning (outcome) at some time in the future for patients with diabetes. In contrast, use of the admissions per 1,000 patients measure provides no evidence-based link between a higher or lower admission rate nor an improved outcome for the patient.

An important issue to consider is the direction in which the measure should move for improvement: in what direction is "goodness?" Is more better, or is less better? Norms are found on the left side of the spectrum, and standards are found on the right. Norms are a measure of what most people do most of the time, or at least at the time of measurement, and do not imply that what people are (or were) doing is right, good, wrong, or bad. Norms are simply a measure of what is (or was). For "use" measures, norms provide a comparison. For example, the admissions-per-1,000-patients measure is compared with fee-for-service norms, managed care norms, Medicare norms, and other norms.

In contrast, clinical performance measures are compared with a standard. A standard is a declaration of what should be done, and frequently articulates the minimum behavior expected. In the diabetes example, it is expected that patients with diabetes will receive at least one eye examination per year. Therefore, a theoretical standard can exist in which 100% of patients with diabetes receive a yearly eye examination. However, in day-to-day living, such an achievement is unlikely. What is more likely is the calculation of an achievable benchmark. This benchmark is the manifestation of "best practice."

The input to clinical performance measures is data. Measures on the left of the spectrum are fed by administrative data. As measures move to the right, they require additional data sources. Enrollment data allow for improved demographic factors and provide a sense of how long a patient has been available to receive care. Pharmacy data is a useful adjunct to clinical data in identifying patients with a particular clinical condition. For example, patients who use insulin most likely have a diagnosis of diabetes. Pharmacy data can also form the basis for a clinical performance measure, such as the use of beta-blockers after an acute myocardial infarction. Data from laboratory results take the clinical performance measures to a new level of refinement. For example, patients with diabetes whose condition is "under control" may need an eye examination every two years instead of every year. To determine whether a patient's condition is in or out of control, the patient's blood glucose level, or hemoglobin A1c (HbA1c) value is needed. Such data would help "clean up" the denominator of the clinical performance measure. In the diabetes example, only patients whose condition was "out-of-control" would be included in the denominator for a measure of yearly eye examinations.

Lastly, as measures move from left to right, they become more valuable to physicians in managing patients. Telling a physician that his or her admission rate per 1,000 patients is too high or too low is meaningless. Physicians deal with individuals and not heterogeneous groups of 1,000 people. Therefore, the more accurately a CPM measures the process of care that is under the control of the physician, and the more closely it can be related to individual patients, the more useful it is to the physician.

Techniques for Reporting

Data collection and analysis efforts are futile if the information generated from these undertakings is not used. For managerial decisionmaking, the vast quantities of available data must be generated in ways that highlight important findings and trends. Determining the most effective means of presenting research findings generally requires presenting the data in multiple ways and refining promising approaches until the findings are clear.[30]

One method of presenting quality data is to capture multiple dimensions, including cost dimensions such as functional health status, satisfaction, cost, and clinical outcomes. Such a display assists managers and clinicians in analyzing the delivery process and measuring the value of care for patient populations to determine how to improve outcomes and lower the costs. The display focuses attention on issues beyond the immediate clinical problem. The approach is holistic in that it considers patient expectations, overall costs, and the impact of treatment choices on the patient's physical, mental, and social functioning.

A second method of presenting quality data is through control charts, which are visual instruments that monitor quality control. Control charts provide a visual means of observing activity that falls outside the normal range by plotting P values for trend data. Control charts are essentially a methodology for detecting statistically significant changes, and they include a baseline average and control limits. These control limits serve as alarm values; a performance-measure point that falls outside of the control limit is considered a significant event. Identifying such an event alerts management to the need for investigation and action.[31]

Organizational Capacity

The organizational capacity to initiate and sustain quality improvement is increasingly recognized as a critical success factor. *Crossing the Quality Chasm: A New Health Care System for the 21st Century* calls for a renewed commitment to evidence-based medicine, to a systems approach, and to patient centeredness.[10] Central to a systems view of health care delivery is the recognition that health care professionals work in an environment that must be designed to facilitate their work. Figure 5–5, adapted from *Crossing the Quality Chasm*, highlights the central role of organizational factors.

Shortell provided a framework for thinking about these organizational factors by documenting that certain levels of organizational capacity need to be in place for quality improvement to be initiated and sustained.[32] He grouped factors into four dimensions: strategic, cultural, technical, and structural (see Table 5–2). Substantial compliance in each "bucket" has different consequences. If strategic factors, such as senior-management commitment and involvement, are not in place, no substantial progress will be made. The absence of fundamental cultural changes will result in only

Figure 5–5   Quality and Organizational Capacity Needs

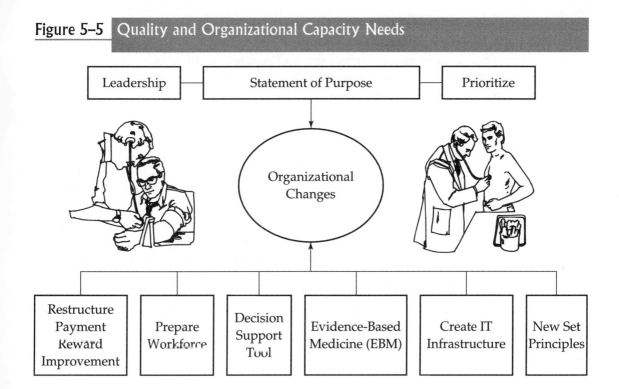

Table 5–2   Impact on Quality Improvement

Strategic	×	Cultural	×	Technical	×	Structural	=	Results
0		1		1		1		No significant results on anything really important
1		0		1		1		Small, temporary effects; no lasting impact
1		1		0		1		Frustration and false starts
1		1		1		0		Inability to capture the learning and spread it throughout the organization
0		1		1		1		Lasting organization-wide impact

0 = absent; 1 = fully present

Source: Shortell S. Assessing the impact of continuous quality improvement on clinical practice: What it will take to accelerate progress. *The Milbank Quarterly.* 1998;76(4).

small and temporary improvements. If technical factors, such as staff training, are not dealt with, false starts and frustration will result. Finally, if structural factors, such as the appropriate committee structures and an information infrastructure to support quality measurement, are not in place, disseminated and sustained improvement will not occur. Shortell maintained that sustained and lasting improvement will only be achieved if all factors are in place.

Evaluating an Information Infrastructure

The evaluation of an information system should focus on technical efficiency and the ability to meet the needs of the end user. To achieve technical efficiency, the components of the information infrastructure should be examined: (1) to determine what is expected, and (2) to explore how well the infrastructure is performing. To satisfy the end user, the evaluation should center on whether the needs and perceptions of consumers, physicians, organizations, and governments are being met.

On the technical side, the following types of questions need to be asked: Have key data sources been accessed? Are standards in place for data content, structure, and coding? Is information sufficiently detailed to answer critical questions? Are data transmitted among organizations with relative ease, and do the systems interact well? Are data stored in the most appropriate ways to facilitate extraction and analysis? Are the systems user-friendly? Are reports generated with ease and speed? Are the data current and accurate? Is the Internet interface user-friendly? Are the data secure? Are multiple firewalls used? How difficult is it for an unauthorized person to access the data?

For the end user, answers to the following questions are important: Is the investment cost-effective? Is the system efficient? Are the data sources adequate to answer key questions? To what extent does the system contribute to the ability to measure and promote quality? Is the investment leading to increases in user satisfaction? Are outcomes improved? What is the return on investment? Is practice variation reduced? Are the information and communication needs of patients, physicians, and managers being met?

Barriers to Development of a Health Information Infrastructure

Although an electronic information infrastructure holds much promise for improving the quality of health care services, the rapid development of information technology faces many technical, financial, and political barriers. Technical barriers include the complexity, decentralization, and fragmentation of the health care system, as well as the lack of standards for terminology, coding, and data transmission. Financial obstacles include the relative absence of payment incentives tied to quality measurement, the inability to demonstrate a convincing return on investment for large information technology undertakings, the low capital investment in information technology, and the fear among health care organizations of exchanging information with competing providers. A variety of political barriers also exist, such as industry regulation issues, intellectual property issues, and concerns about confidentiality and privacy.

The highly complex and fragmented nature of the U.S. health care system hampers the ability to collect and analyze data within and across organizations. Data collection and analysis processes entail combining data from various sources and making comparisons using different information systems and processes. Measuring the quality of care requires access to a wide range of information from varying sources. However, health care programs, plans, and providers may use different software packages for different requirements (e.g., claims processing, utilization management, and provider credentialing); and basic data, such as patient identifiers, may vary between health plans and sometimes even between different providers within a plan. Moreover, many providers are not part of large health care systems with high-powered information networks. The U.S. health care system is highly decentralized; 40% of practices have just one physician, and 80% have fewer than 10 physicians. Of the approximately 5,000 hospitals in the United States, an estimated 3,500 belong to a network.[10]

Little consistency in standards for terminology, data coding, or data transmission exists across providers or vendors. Although some standards developed by organizations accredited by the American National Standards Institute (ANSI) are in fairly wide use, much variation exists because many organizations modify these standards for their own purposes. Moreover, vendors for each clinical system often have unique classification systems. This lack of consistency presents an important barrier to an information infrastructure for improving quality measurement, because the absence of uniform data standards impedes the aggregation of data from local to national levels. Measuring and interpreting outcomes, providing continuous quality improvement, and allocating limited resources to optimize quality and effectiveness require comparable data.[13]

Currently, a main obstacle to information technology development in the health care field is the low expenditure on these systems compared with that in other industries. For example, the expenditure on information technology is $543 per employee in the health sector, whereas it is $12,666 per employee among security brokers. Health care ranks 38 out of 58 industries in its investment in information technology.[10]

One reason for this low expenditure may be that the return on the investment is difficult to prove. Another reason may be that investments in large data warehouses, the development of which is often costly and time consuming, have failed to meet expectations.[27, 29] Investment in quality improvement technology may be limited in part because payment incentives do not encourage it.[2] Fear of sharing information with competitors may also slow progress toward development of an integrated information infrastructure because providers may believe that they are jeopardizing their competitive position. Further, providers may not want to change their data management systems to accommodate more standardized ones because they believe that the cost of doing so is unnecessary.[3]

In the political arena, data privacy and confidentiality issues are highly visible. Another important policy issue that may present an information technology roadblock is regulation. For example, the question of whether clinical decision software should be regulated as a medical device by the Food and Drug Administration has been under debate. Other concerns relate to intellectual property (copyright and patent) issues and liability.[33]

● A Case Study of Disease Management Interventions

A variety of health care organizations could be used in a case study to illustrate the use of disease management interventions (e.g., employer, health plan, integrated delivery system, or physician group). In this case study, a health plan is used, and the health plan administrators are aware that disease management interventions ensure appropriate utilization as outlined by clinical practice guidelines. By managing certain clinical conditions using disease management techniques, the plan administrators hope to better understand what the plan pays for services, how to improve care, and how to maintain or lower costs. These disease management techniques can be used to:

- Assure that primary prevention interventions are being used in the healthy segment of the enrollee population
- Identify which secondary prevention interventions to use in the segment of the population with existing conditions
- Identify which tertiary prevention interventions to use in the segment of the enrollee population with extensive disease

In this example, the health plan administration intends to focus on enrollees who are the most ill, whose care will cost them the most in the coming year, and who have a condition for which disease management improves with the use of evidence-based interventions. Some specific acute and chronic conditions that are high-cost, prevalent, and amenable to disease management interventions are asthma, chronic obstructive pulmonary disease, coronary artery disease, depression, diabetes, heart failure, hypertension, lower back pain, otitis media, nonstreptococcal pharyngitis, and sinusitis. Here, disease management interventions are effective because of the availability of two critical factors for successful disease management interventions—evidence-based clinical practice guidelines and clinical performance measures.

The health plan's analysis involves:

1. Grouping all enrollees into cost cohorts for the current year
2. Identifying enrollees, within each current-year cohort, who are predicted to be the most expensive to care for in the coming year
3. Identifying which of those enrollees (i.e., those predicted to be the most expensive to care for in the coming year) have a condition amenable to disease management
4. Risk-stratifying these enrollees with this condition
5. Determining the amount of evidence-based services that the enrollees received for the condition in the current year
6. Determining which enrollees received few or none of the evidence-based interventions
7. Determining which of the enrollees have the highest opportunity for disease management intervention

This analytical approach allows the plan to identify:

- Enrollees whose care is predicted to be expensive in the coming year
- Enrollees who have the most severe form of the condition
- The conditions for which evidence-based interventions exist
- The frequency of the interventions required for each identified enrollee
- Disease management techniques that are amenable to the use of the evidence-based interventions

Here, diabetes serves as a clinical example for the approach. Methodologies, such as Diagnostic Cost Groups (DCG), Medstat's Episode Grouper (MEG), and Study Group Subsets (SGS), are used to accomplish the following analytic steps:

Step 1: The health plan groups enrollees by cost of care for the current year using DCGs.

Step 2: DCGs provide a method for predicting the costs of care for these populations in the coming year.

Step 3: Within the group of enrollees, the plan identifies enrollees with diabetes using a method that groups enrollees into clinically unique categories. Medstat Episode Grouper (MEG) places these high-cost enrollees into a diabetes episode and further risk-stratifies them into three integer stages (1, 2, or 3), depending on the severity of their diabetes. If needed, MEG can also divide each integer stage into as many as nine substages for finer stratification.

Step 4: The health plan determines which evidence-based interventions for diabetes were provided to enrollees with the most severe diabetes. An example of an evidence-based intervention for diabetes is hemoglobin A1c (HbA1c) testing, which some clinical practice guidelines recommend performing quarterly. The diabetes MEG is used to identify the denominator population, and the numerator consists of enrollees who have had 4 HbA1c tests during the year. This measure provides the rate of HbA1c tests for the population with diabetes and a list of enrollees who have, and who have not, had four tests annually. However, it does not reveal the distribution of the four HbA1c tests throughout the four quarters of the year.

Step 5: SGS allows the health plan to identify each enrollee who received four HbA1c tests during the past year and to list the number of tests that they received each quarter. The health plan disease management program may contact any enrollee who did not receive an HbA1c test each quarter, the enrollee's primary care provider, or both, to alert them to the ideal testing schedule.

References

1. Chassin MR. Is health care ready for six sigma quality? *The Milbank Quarterly*. 1998;76(4):565–591, 610.

2. Chassin MR, Gavin RW, and the National Roundtable on Health Care Quality. The urgent need to improve health care quality. *JAMA*. 1998;280(11):1000–1005.

3. President's Advisory Commission on Consumer Protection in the Health Care Industry. *Quality First: Better Health Care for All Americans*. Rockville, Md: Agency for Healthcare Research and Quality; 1998.

4. Joint Commission on Accreditation of Healthcare Organizations (JCAHO). Available at: http://www.jcaho.org.

5. National Committee for Quality Assurance. Available at: http://www.ncqa.org/.

6. National Quality Forum. Available at: http://www.qualityforum.org/.

7. The Leapfrog Group. Available at: http://www.leapfroggroup.org

8. Institute of Medicine. *To Err Is Human: Building a Safer Health System*. Washington, DC: Institute of Medicine; 1999.

9. Institute of Medicine. *Envisioning the National Health Care Quality Report*. Washington, DC: Institute of Medicine; 2001.

10. Institute of Medicine. *Crossing the Quality Chasm: A New Health System for the 21st Century*. Washington, DC: Institute of Medicine; 2001.

11. Sackett DL, Straus SE, Richardson WS, et al. *Evidence-Based Medicine: How to Practice and Teach EBM*. 2nd ed. London, England: Churchill Livingstone; 2000.

12. Bates D. Effect of computerized physician order entry and a team intervention of serious medication errors. *JAMA*. 1998;280(15):1311–1316.

13. Computer-Based Patient Record Institute (CPRI). Action Plan for Development of Health Data Standards, Action Plan for Addressing Confidentiality and Security Issues in Implementing Computer-Based Patient Record Systems, Action Plan for Implementing a Unique Health Identifier; 2001. Available at: http://www.himss.org/asp/cpritoolkit_homepage.asp.

14. Bakken S. An informatics infrastructure is essential for evidence-based practice. *J Am Med Inform Assoc.* 2001;8(3):199–201.

15. Chute C, Cohn SP, Campbell KE, et al. The content coverage of clinical classifications. *Journal of the American Medical Informatics Association.* 1996;3(3):224–233.

16. Coenen A, Marin, HF, Park HA, Bakken S. Collaborative efforts for representing nursing concepts in computer-based systems. *Journal of the American Medical Informatics Association.* 2001;8(3):202–211.

17. Centers for Disease Control (CDC). Available at: http://www.cdc.gov/nchs/icd9.htm.

18. Unified Medical Language System (UMLS). Available at: http://www.nlm.nih.gov/research/umls/.

19. McDonald CJ. Need for standards in heath information. *Health Affairs* 1998;17(6):44–46.

20. The Regenstrief Institute. Logical Observation Identifiers, Names, and Codes. Available at: http://www.regenstrief.org/loinc/.

21. Institute of Medicine. Patient Safety Achieving a New Standard for Care. Philip Aspden, Janet M. Corrigan, Julie Wolcott & Shari M. Erickson, Eds. Washington, DC: Institute of Medicine; 2004.

22. Personal communication, HIPAA compliance officer, MEDSTAT on HIPAA standards.

23. Cimino JJ. Beyond the superhighway: Exploiting the Internet with medical informatics. *Journal of the American Medical Informatics Association.* 1997;4(4):279–284.

24. Goldsmith J. The Internet and managed care: A new wave of innovation. *Health Affairs.* 2000;19(1):42–56.

25. Kaplan B, Brennan PF, Dowling AF, Friedman CP, Peel V. Towards an informatics research agenda. *Journal of the American Medical Informatics Association.* 2001;8(3):235–241.

26. Niedzwiecki P, Priest SL, Pivnicny VC, Ruffino BC. Leveraging HIPAA to support consumer empowerment. *Journal of Healthcare Information Management.* 2000;14(4):95–104.

27. Bush D. Why is data warehousing failing us? *Managed Healthcare News.* 2000;16(6).

28. Breen C, Rodrigues LM. Implementing a data warehouse at Inglis Innovative Services. *Journal of Healthcare Information Management Systems Society.* 2001;15(2)87–97.

29. Ramick DC. Data warehousing in disease management programs. *Journal of Healthcare Information Management Systems Society.* 2001;15(2):99–105.

30. Tufte E. *The Visual Display of Quantitative Information.* Cheshire, Conn: Graphics Press; 2001.

31. National Institute of Standards and Technology. NIST/SEMATECH e-Handbook of Statistical Methods. Available at: http://www.itl.nist.gov/div898/handbook/. Accessed on July 13, 2004.

32. Shortell S. Assessing the impact of continuous quality improvement on clinical practice: What it will take to accelerate progress. *The Milbank Quarterly.* 1998;76(4):593–624, 625.

33. Moran D. Health information policy: On preparing for the next war. *Health Affairs.* 1998;17(6):9–22.

Chapter 6

LEGAL AND ETHICAL ISSUES IN MEDICAL QUALITY MANAGEMENT

Joseph A. Mislove, JD, MBA
Jeffrey Zale, MD, MPH

Introduction to Part I: Legal Issues

The first section of this chapter describes the basic legal framework for medical quality management, and the second part outlines some basic ethical principles. The purpose of both sections is to provide a working knowledge of each subject that will be relevant to the rest of the curriculum.

Any discipline must operate within an established set of legal and ethical standards, and medical quality management is no different. In fact, medical quality managers should carefully follow these standards for two reasons. First, quality managers strive to identify, maintain, and promote practices that lead to quality care, and change practices and behavior when necessary. Those who promote the quality of medical practice among peers must have credibility and the tools of persuasion, especially if they are to promote professional behavior change. A solid legal and ethical footing provides the framework in which credible and persuasive quality management activities can occur. Second, the legal and ethical framework for medical quality management reflects societal preferences on how to balance the interests of patients, practitioners, institutional providers, health plans, regulatory agencies, and the general public. Legal and ethical standards help to ensure that these preferences are honored.

Modern health care consists of a number of administrative and financial activities that support the delivery of care. The legal motivation for many activities that are ancillary to direct patient care often involves the fact that a law or an accreditation standard requires the activity, and that the activity helps manage the liability risk for a bad outcome. In the case of medical quality management, both of these reasons apply.

Regulatory and Accreditation Requirements for Medical Quality Management

Hospitals and other institutional providers are often required to perform medical quality management under the terms of a state license. For example, a hospital licensed by the State of Arizona must establish, implement, and document an ongoing medical quality management program.[1] A hospital in Illinois must have rules that are consistent with state statute on granting, limiting, renewing, or denying medical staff membership.[2]

Medicare and Medicaid programs also require that hospitals perform medical quality management. To receive payment for services under Medicare or Medicaid, hospitals must comply with the conditions of participation set forth in the regulations. One condition provides that a hospital must have "an effective hospital-wide quality assurance program to evaluate the provision of patient care."[3]

Most hospitals also follow accreditation standards of the Joint Commission on the Accreditation of Healthcare Organizations (JCAHO); hospitals must meet certain Medicare requirements if they are JCAHO-accredited.[4] The JCAHO standards, along with the Medicare Conditions of Participation, set detailed requirements on how to organize and perform medical quality management, which include credentialing, peer review, and organizational performance improvement.

Health plans are similarly required to perform medical quality management under the insurance or health care laws of some states. New York, for example, will not issue a certificate of authority to any health maintenance organization unless "acceptable procedures have been established to monitor the quality of care provided by the plan."[5]

At the federal level, a health plan participating in the Medicare + Choice program "must have . . . an ongoing quality assessment and performance improvement program that meets applicable requirements [set forth in the regulation]."[6] Similarly, under federal Medicaid regulations that states must follow as of June 2003, a state's contract with a health plan must require that the plan "have an ongoing quality assessment and performance improvement program for the services it furnishes to its enrollees."[7]

As indicated above, most hospitals and health plans are required to engage in medical quality management by state licensing laws, federal health care program requirements, or accreditation standards. As seen below, liability issues also provide motivation for organizations to perform medical quality management.

Risk Management Incentives to Conduct Medical Quality Management

As seen in the negligence cases described in the following paragraphs, courts have held hospitals and health plans liable for the care provided by independent practitioners. The cases involve physicians who were not employed by the organization but who were independent contractors of the medical staff or network. As a result, hospitals and health plans should promote quality physician care through credentialing and peer review of independent practitioners.

Most of the hospital negligence cases in this area focus on controlling quality through the physicians authorized to practice at the facility. For example, one court held that a hospital must prevent an independent contractor physician that it knows or should know is incompetent from practicing at the facility.[8] Another court found that a hospital had a duty to make sure that its independent contractor physicians were competent enough to perform surgery.[9]

Not surprisingly, courts hold health plans that own and operate their own clinics (staff models) responsible for the care provided by independent consulting physicians.[10] Health plans that assemble a network of independent physicians who practice out of their own offices are also legally responsible for selecting competent professionals. The courts have decided that a health plan limits an enrollee's choice of physicians to those the plan has selected for the network and requires or encourages the enrollee to use those physicians, which creates the impression that the health plan is the source of care.[11]

A recent Florida case illustrates how an organization contracting for physician services can be held accountable for the quality of an independent physician's care. Susan Villazon was a member of an HMO. Sadly, Ms. Villazon died from untreated cancer. Her husband sued the primary care physician, a doctor who participated in the HMO's network of independent contracted practitioners. The husband claimed that the HMO was "vicariously liable," meaning that it was responsible for the negligent acts of the physician, even though the physician ran his own independent practice. The Florida Supreme Court found that the HMO had the right to control how physicians in its network rendered medical services to members. The potential for control was enough, according to the Court, to allow the claim to proceed against the HMO for the allegedly negligent actions of its contracted physician.

Although physicians of the past, in the traditional pattern of American life, may have constituted distinct independent businesses and independent centers of occupation and profession, the HMO concept has substantially altered that model in a manner that the legal system cannot simply ignore. A visit to a private office of a completely independent physician may now be more an historical event than current reality.[12] As a result, with increasing frequency, the legal system finds that HMOs, like hospitals, have a duty to select competent physicians and are responsible for the quality of care delivered.

Negligence cases, coupled with licensing and Medicare requirements, provide ample reason for a hospital or health plan to monitor the quality of care provided by physicians authorized to treat patients and enrollees. The implementation of the risk management strategy is driven, in large part, by the legal framework described below.

Legal Responsibility for Conducting Medical Quality Management

Medicare and many states hold the governing body of a hospital, usually a board of directors or trustees, ultimately responsible for the quality of care at the facility. The medical staff, however, must perform the actual medical quality management activities.

Under Medicare, for example, hospitals are required to have "an organized medical staff" that, among other things, must be "accountable to the governing body for the quality of medical care provided to patients."[13] In Arizona, the governing body of each licensed hospital must require physicians with privileges at the facility to form committees to review the professional practices in the hospital.[14]

Many owners and sponsors of health plans follow the hospital model and place responsibility for medical quality management with a governing body. The governing body, in turn, delegates quality management activities to a chief medical officer or to various committees. This structure is encouraged through accreditation standards.

State insurance regulators indirectly make the health plan governing body responsible for medical quality management by making an HMO or utilization review license conditional on an annual quality management or improvement plan. The governing body is then accountable for the plan's implementation, as it is for all conditions of licensure.

Legal Protections for Conducting Peer Review: Confidentiality and Immunity

Peer review in medical quality management is the process by which physicians evaluate the qualifications of other physicians (i.e., their peers) who have applied for privileges to practice at a hospital or other health care facility, or for credentials to participate in a network maintained by a health plan. Peer review also involves the process through which a physician's actions are reviewed by peers for possible corrective action, discipline, or revocation of privileges or credentials. From the public's perspective, peer review improves medical care by subjecting practicing physicians to supervision and corrective action, including adverse actions on privileges and credentials, by their fellow health professionals.

Historically, two legal actions have threatened the effectiveness of—and physician participation in—medical quality management activities. One such action is the discovery process of a lawsuit, in which access to quality management documents is sought to find potentially damaging information. For example, a candid written response by a physician under investigation, or a report by a physician reviewer for a quality management investigation, might be very attractive to a plaintiff who is suing the physician for medical malpractice.

The other legal action involves lawsuits brought by physicians against the organization for its quality management activities, or against the peer review committee for its actions against them, such as denial of practice privileges or revocation, or limitation of privileges or credentials. Either action, whether it actually occurs or is simply possible, reduces physicians' willingness to participate and to communicate candidly in medical quality management activities as a reviewer or as a person under review. This "chilling effect" can potentially limit the quality management information-gathering and review processes.

In response, lawmakers have passed "peer review confidentiality" laws to protect from discovery information obtained or developed during medical quality management activities in medical malpractice and other lawsuits. Lawmakers have also passed "peer review immunity" laws to protect physicians from lawsuits filed for adverse privilege or credentialing actions. Many of these laws contain conditions that medical quality management activities and participants must follow if the protections of the laws are to apply. In addition, provisions in the laws, and in the court decisions interpreting them, identify circumstances in which the protection provided through confidentiality or immunity may not apply.

Confidentiality of Peer Review Proceedings

Confidentiality provisions are found in state peer review statutes. Such statutes typically protect the confidentiality of information and documents used by the peer review component (usually a committee) of medical quality management. In other words, the documents or information used for peer review are generally not subject to discovery or subpoena.

For example, in Pennsylvania, the "proceedings and records of a review committee" are not "subject to discovery or introduction into evidence in any civil action against a professional" that arises out of the events reviewed by the committee.[15] In Arizona, the information and records of actions and proceedings of a quality assurance process are confidential and are not subject to subpoena or orders to produce.[16] There are, however, notable exceptions to these protections, as outlined below.

The purpose of confidentiality provisions is to encourage physicians to engage in peer review with candor and to alleviate concerns that criticism of another physician's conduct will support a claim in a malpractice lawsuit rather than improve the quality of medical care. The American Medical Association (AMA) has recognized the importance of confidentiality to effective peer review as a matter of policy.[17] The AMA's position supports the quality management activities in hospitals, especially the oversight of physicians by fellow members of the medical staff, many of whom are AMA members or follow its professional principles. Similarly, when interpreting peer review confidentiality statutes, the "courts have recognized that the confidentiality of peer review committee proceedings is essential to achieve complete investigation and review of medical care . . . [and that peer review] deliberations would terminate if they were subject to the discovery process."[18]

Because confidentiality laws are intended to promote effective peer review, there are relatively simple conditions under the statutes to obtain their protection. In Pennsylvania, the confidentiality provisions apply to a committee that engages health care professionals to evaluate the quality and efficiency of medical services by other health care professionals for any of the following purposes: to improve quality of care, to reduce morbidity and mortality, and to establish and enforce guidelines that are designed to keep health care costs within reason.[19]

In Arizona, the information and records of actions and proceedings are confidential and not subject to subpoena or orders to produce, so long as the quality review process is formally adopted by the health care organization and follows written standards. The confidentiality protection then extends to activities of the health care organization or any of its committees that investigate the quality of health care or that encourage proper use of health care services and facilities.[20]

The protections offered by the confidentiality laws do not apply in all circumstances. In Pennsylvania, documents or records otherwise available from other sources are not immune from discovery.[21] In Arizona, confidentiality provisions do not apply in proceedings before a state licensing agency, which means that the state agency can subpoena the information and records of actions and proceedings of a peer review committee.[22] However, the privileged committee information is kept confidential by the state agency. In addition, a health care provider who files a lawsuit against a health care organization can obtain peer review committee records about his or her own case.

A number of court cases have allowed access to peer review information on the basis of an exception to a state confidentiality statue. For example, in *Hayes v. Mercy Health Corporation*,[23] the Pennsylvania Supreme Court held that the confidentiality provisions did not apply to a physician challenging his own peer review process. In *Virmani v. Novant Health, Inc.*,[24] the court granted Dr. Virmani access to the hospital's peer review records of all physicians reviewed for any reason during the previous 20 years to assess his claim of discrimination. Finally, in *Public Citizen, Inc. v. Dept.*

of Health and Human Services,[25] a federal court held that the agency overseeing the Medicare program must disclose the results of an investigation into the quality of care received by a Medicare beneficiary. Such investigations are performed by a Quality Improvement Organization (formerly Peer Review Organization) under contract with the federal government, pursuant to the confidentiality provisions of the federal Peer Review Improvement Act. Medicare regulations permitted release of investigation results only with the consent of the physician under review. The court found that such regulations contradicted the federal statute under which a Quality Improvement Organization must inform the Medicare beneficiary of the final disposition of the complaint.[26]

Immunity of Peer Reviewers

Both federal and state laws grant immunity from damages to physicians, hospitals, and other organizations for actions arising from peer review processes. In other words, if a peer review immunity law applies, a hospital and the members of its medical staff peer review committee cannot be sued by a physician disgruntled over the loss of hospital privileges through peer review.

Peer review immunity laws are passed "for the express purpose of encouraging good faith peer review . . . [and their] goal is to foster an environment in which health care professionals will be encouraged to engage in good faith evaluation of their peers by limiting participants' potential liability."[27] In fact, the rationale for peer review immunity was so important that Congress, in its statutory findings in the *Health Care Quality Improvement Act of 1986* (HCQIA), declared that the threat of monetary damages "unreasonably discourages physicians from participating in effective peer review," resulting in an "overriding national need to provide incentive and protection [through immunity] for physicians engaging in effective professional peer review."[28]

Arizona's peer review immunity statute, like those in many states, provides that no organization or individual involved in carrying out peer review or related disciplinary duties is liable for damages to any person whose privileges are suspended, limited, or revoked.[29] Some states, like Pennsylvania, condition immunity on the exercise of due care or absence of malice while performing peer review.[30]

Federal law, in the form of the HCQIA, is extremely important in peer review immunity because it applies nationally. In addition, if a state law allows a lawsuit to be brought for damages where HCQIA does not, the HCQIA immunity provisions would likely prevail under federal preemption. The HCQIA is also important in other aspects of medical quality management because of its fair hearing and data-bank reporting provisions. Each of these provisions, in addition to the conditions for and exceptions to peer review immunity, is discussed in detail below.

Conditions for Peer Review Immunity Under the Health Care Quality Improvement Act

As indicated above, the HCQIA, described in federal statutes 42 U.S.C. §§ 11101 through 11152, protects institutions and individuals engaged in peer review. The HCQIA provides limited immunity in the form of protection from damages under federal and state law for "professional review actions" by "professional review bodies" and the individuals who take part in such actions, including a member or staff person of the professional review body, a person under contract with the professional review body, and any other person who participates in or assists the professional review body.[31] To receive immunity protection under the HCQIA, a professional review action must meet all of the following conditions:[32]

1. The action must adversely affect the clinical privileges of a physician and be based on professional conduct or competence.

2. The adverse action must be imposed with the reasonable belief that it furthers quality health care.

3. A reasonable effort to obtain the facts of the matter must be undertaken before the adverse action is imposed.

4. The adverse action is imposed after the physician affected by it receives adequate notice and an opportunity for a hearing that adheres to certain procedures.

The HCQIA presumes that a peer review process meets the preceding standards "unless the presumption is rebutted by a preponderance of the evidence."[33] Thus, a physician challenging peer review "bears the burden of proving that the peer review process was not reasonable."[34] Whether the process is reasonable or not is evaluated under an objective standard; that is, would a reasonable person have reached a similar peer review decision based on the information from the investigation?[35]

For example, a hospital was held to be immune from liability under the HCQIA; the decision to revoke a physician's privileges was based on a review of 22 incident reports involving the physician's loss of temper during surgery, breaking of the sterile field, and failure to take and document patient histories before sedation. On review, the court found that the peer reviewers reasonably believed that they were furthering quality health care, and their actions were clearly warranted by the facts.[36]

Even under the presumption and objective standard described above, which favors the organization and participants conducting peer review, some physicians have successfully argued that a peer review process was not reasonable. For example, an obstetrician used an expert who had reviewed all of his cases within a six-month period to show that the hospital's review of only two cases was not a reasonable peer review process.[37]

In another case, a physician was able to overcome immunity and maintain a damages claim against a hospital by showing that it had revoked his privileges because he had reported to outside agencies concerns over quality of care as well as conflicts at the hospital. In other words, the peer review action did not objectively further quality health care because the doctor had no quality issues and lost his privileges as a result of his whistle-blowing activities, not from professional incompetence.[38]

Fair Hearing Procedures Under the Health Care Quality Improvement Act

The HCQIA requires that notice and hearing procedures must be followed if immunity is to be maintained for an adverse peer review action. As a result, the HCQIA "fair hearing" procedures, as they are sometimes called, are often the framework for the appeal policy that a hospital or other health care organization offers a physician aggrieved by a peer review decision.

Essentially, 42 U.S.C. § 11112(b) requires that the physician subject to the adverse action receive notice of the proposed action to be taken, a summary of his or her rights to be afforded at the hearing, and adequate notice of the hearing. The physician's rights at the hearing, set forth in § 11112(b)(3), include the right to: (1) representation by counsel; (2) have a record made of the proceedings; (3) call and cross-examine witnesses; (4) submit a written closing statement; and (5) receive a final written decision by the health care organization.

The HCQIA, however, also provides that the failure of a review body to meet these five conditions exactly does not automatically constitute a failure to meet the standards necessary for immunity under § 11112(a)(3).[39] Instead, the test is whether the notice and hearing procedures were adequate or fair to the physician under the circumstances.[40]

Data Bank Reporting Under HCQIA: The National Practitioner Data Bank

The National Practitioner Data Bank (NPDB) was established under the HCQIA as an alert or flagging system of information about a practitioner's licensure, privilege, and malpractice history. The information in the NPDB is intended to supplement other information obtained for the credentialing process and to identify aspects of a practitioner's licensure, privilege, or malpractice history that may warrant additional inquiry. The NPDB supports the HCQIA in restricting the ability of incompetent physicians, dentists, and other health care professionals to move to another state without disclosing previous malpractice or adverse actions, such as a denial, loss, or restriction of a license, clinical privilege, professional society membership, or ability to participate in Medicare or Medicaid.[41]

The reporting provisions appear in the federal statutes along with the other HCQIA provisions.[42] However, regulations that govern how the NPDB operates are found at 45 Code of Federal Regulations (C.F.R.) Part 60, which is reflected in citations 43–47.

Reporting information under the NPDB is limited to medical malpractice payers, state licensing medical boards and dental examiners, professional societies with formal peer review, hospitals, and health care organizations. A health care organization is one that provides health care services and engages in professional review activity through either a formal peer review process for the purpose of furthering quality health care or a committee of that organization with the same purpose.[43] The regulation also provides that a health care organization could include: (1) a health maintenance organization that is either licensed by the state or qualified by the Department of Health and Human Services as a health maintenance organization; or (2) any group or prepaid medical or dental practice that engages in professional review activity, as outlined in the definition.

Any organization that pays a medical malpractice claim for the benefit of a physician, dentist, or other health care practitioner must report the claim to the NPDB if the payment is in settlement of, or in satisfaction in whole or in part of, a written claim or a judgment against the practitioner. A payment is not reportable if it is made as a result of a suit or claim solely against an organization (e.g., a hospital, clinic, or group practice) that does not identify an individual practitioner.

To be reportable, the medical malpractice payment must be limited to an exchange of money and must be the result of a written complaint or claim demanding monetary payment for damages for a practitioner's provision of or failure to provide a health care service.[44]

State medical and dental boards must report certain actions taken against the licenses of physicians or dentists by hospitals and other eligible health care organizations. Specifically, such boards must report revocation, suspension, censure, reprimand, probation, and surrender of licensure. Any revisions to the adverse licensure action must also be reported.[45]

Hospitals and other eligible health care organizations *must* report adverse actions on clinical privileges of a physician or dentist and *may* report such an action against a licensed health care practitioner other than a physician or dentist. The reporting obligation is triggered by a professional review action that adversely affects clinical privileges for more than 30 days. Additionally, a hospital or other health care organization must report a physician or dentist who voluntarily surrenders or restricts clinical privileges while under investigation or in return for not conducting an investigation or professional review action.[46]

A professional society *must* report to the NPDB any professional review action related to professional competence or conduct that adversely affects the membership of a physician or dentist. A professional society of health professionals other than physicians and dentists *may* report adverse actions taken against a member.[47]

Information reported to the NPDB is confidential and may not be disclosed except as specified in the NPDB regulations. Specifically, 45 C.F.R. § 60.10 requires that hospitals must request information from the data bank concerning a physician, dentist, or health care practitioner on initial application for clinical privileges and every two years thereafter. Under 45 C.F.R. § 60.11, the NPDB will make information in its data bank available to the following:

1. A hospital that requests information concerning a physician, dentist, or other health care practitioner who is on the medical staff or has clinical privileges

2. A physician, dentist, or other health care practitioner requesting information about him- or herself

3. A medical or dental board, or other state licensing board

4. A health care organization that has entered or may be entering into employment, affiliation, or clinical privilege relationships with a physician, dentist, or other health care practitioner

5. An attorney who has filed a medical practice action against a hospital, and who requests information regarding a specific physician, dentist, or other health care provider who is also named in the action

6. A health care organization conducting a professional review activity

7. A person or organization who requests information in a form that does not identify any particular health care organization, physician, dentist, or other health care practitioner

A person or organization who receives NPDB information directly or indirectly is subject to 45 C.F.R. § 69.13, which requires that database information remain confidential and that it be used solely with respect to the purpose for which it was provided. Violators of this provision are subject to a federal penalty of up to $10,000 for each violation.

In terms of immunity, the HCQIA, at 42 U.S.C. § 11137 (c), states that no person or organization shall be held liable in any civil action with respect to any report made to the NPDB without knowledge of the falsity of the information contained in the report.

Data Bank Reporting Under HIPAA: The Healthcare Integrity Protection Data Bank

Ten years after the NPDB was created, Congress decided that a comprehensive source of fraud and abuse and other adverse action information on practitioners was needed in addition to the NPDB. Under the Health Insurance Portability and Accountability Act of 1996 (HIPAA), Public Law 104-191, Congress required a second national data bank—The Healthcare Integrity Protection Data Bank (HIPDB)—to receive and disclose the following adverse actions:

1. Civil judgments against a health care provider, supplier, or practitioner (collectively, "Provider") in federal or state court related to the delivery of a health care item or service

2. Federal or state criminal convictions against a Provider related to the delivery of a health care item or service

3. Actions by federal and state Provider licensing and certification agencies

4. Exclusion of a Provider from participation in federal or state health care programs

5. Any other adjudicated actions or decisions established by regulation

The Healthcare Integrity Protection Data Bank operates pursuant to statute 42 U.S.C. § 1320 A-7 E and regulations at 45 C.F.R. §§ 61.1 through 61.16 (collectively, the "HIPDB Laws"). (Information about the HIPDB and the NPDB is also available at *http://www.npdb-hipdb.com*, a web site operated by the federal government.)

The HIPDB Laws make the information in the data bank available to federal and state government agencies and health plans. These organizations may query the HIPDB, although, unlike NPDB, they are not required to do so. Providers may query the HIPDB for information about themselves (known as "self-query"), but not about other providers. Under the HIPDB Laws, federal and state licensing agencies must report certain final adverse licensure actions against providers, such as the revocation or suspension of a license, the right to apply for or renew a license, or a limitation on the scope of practice. Because a principal goal of the HIPDB is to prevent health care fraud and abuse in addition to improving the quality of patient care, an action need not be based necessarily on a physician's clinical competence or conduct to be reportable.

A voluntary surrender of a license or certification is reportable if it occurs after notification of investigation, after a formal official request by a licensing or certification authority, in exchange for a decision by a licensing or certification authority to cease or not conduct an investigation, or in lieu of a disciplinary proceeding. A voluntary surrender for personal reasons, such as retirement or change to inactive status, is not reportable.

The HIPDB Laws also require that federal and state government agencies and health plans must report "other adjudicated actions or decisions." The action or decision must be based on an act or omission that affects or could affect the payment, provision, or delivery of a health care item or service and must include a due process mechanism, such as a formal appeal that is available before the action becomes final.

Actions by federal or state government agencies and panel decisions by health plans that affect clinical privileges are not reportable to the HIPDB, but they are reportable to the NPDB. Under the preamble of the HIPDB Final Rule, however, health plans must report to the HIPDB actions based on quality, as long as a due process mechanism, such as a formal appeal, is available before the action becomes final.

Conclusion to Part I: Legal Issues

The above laws and regulations constitute the legal framework for medical quality management, especially that portion that relies on peer review to improve quality of care by changing clinical practices and behavior and by disciplining and reporting practitioners under certain circumstances. The legal framework reflects society's preference for protecting the public from substandard practitioners over the economic interests of such practitioners, within certain limits of fairness and reason.

Legal considerations, however, are only one portion of the framework for medical quality management. Ethical considerations, which are described in the next section, are important as well.

Introduction to Part II: Ethical Issues

Ethical philosophies and concepts have influenced much current public policy, law, and government regulation. Ethical concepts and discussions have resulted in the genesis, amendment, and consideration of changes to laws and policies in the areas of physician-assisted suicide and health care rationing, for example. The medical malpractice argument of negligence relates to a physician's failure to practice the ethical concepts of beneficence and nonmaleficence. Laws codify correct action, which has a basis in medical ethics. Laws have been written to mandate certain actions by health care professions; for example, the federal Emergency Medical Treatment and Active Labor Act (EMTALA) requires that patients be evaluated and stabilized before being transferred out of an emergency department. The Patient Self Determination Act of 1991 requires Medicare and Medicaid providers (hospitals, nursing homes, hospice programs, and home health agencies) to inform patients, on admission, of their rights to prepare an advance directive, participate in and direct their own health care decisions, and accept or decline medical or surgical treatment.

Availability, accessibility, and acceptability are all attributes of quality health care. Patient-centered care involves basing the medical care on patient desires, wishes, and values, not those of the physician or other health care professional. Patient participation in creating the medical care plan will increase the patients' willingness to adhere to a jointly determined sequence of preventive or therapeutic care. The endpoint is patient autonomy or empowerment. Medical ethics provides a framework for approaching and evaluating medical issues that involve a patient's decisions and rights, while also considering societal values. The issues of assuring this patient autonomy in deciding when to accept or reject therapy or recommendations is an important part of the education of a professional involved with medical quality.

The field of ethics is used to determine "right action" when no laws or policy support or mandate acting in a particular manner. Knowledge of medical ethics is necessary to understand not only the ramifications of health care policy considerations on a macro level, but also the appropriate action on a more micro level in individual health care facilities and in the physician-patient relationship.

This part of the chapter provides a basic understanding of the field of medical ethics and some of the precepts on which it is based. In addition, the function of an ethics consultant, or committee, and the roles that they serve in a health care facility are described. This part of the chapter is divided into the following sections:

1. What is medical ethics?
2. Why is the study of medical ethics relevant to medical professionals?
3. A short history of ethical thought
4. Ethical theories and principles
5. Types of decisions in which ethical decisionmaking may be necessary
6. Examples of how medical ethical principles can be used to show possible alternatives for resolution of ethical issues
7. Ethics committees

What Is Medical Ethics?

Ethics is a branch of philosophy concerned with the relationships between people and the duties or obligations that individuals have to one another and to society in general. It is a way of understanding, examining, and living a moral life. Medical ethics relates these duties or obligations to health care policy, biomedical research, and medical practice. It applies general ethical principles to issues in the medical context. Although the field of medical ethics is relatively new, begun for the most part within the last 100 years, the larger field of ethics or "moral living" has been an area of inquiry for thousands of years. The schools of ethical thought can be distilled into the generally accepted concepts and medical ethics principles described in the following sections.

The Relevance of Medical Ethics to Medical Professionals

Many dilemmas in medical practice require a framework for analysis. Such dilemmas include what to do when: a patient declines necessary medical care; giving informed consent; making end-of-life decisions; providing futile care or heroic measures; and rationing health care resources.

Analyzing an ethical issue is similar to making a clinical diagnosis. Physicians typically start with a differential diagnosis of possibilities, narrow the diagnosis to a single disease, and then choose the treatment that has the greatest likelihood of success. The radiologist views a chest x-ray in a particular manner—first the bones, then the heart, and finally the lungs. A primary care doctor obtains information, first from the history, then from the physical, and finally from specific studies or tests.

The method for analyzing moral dilemmas and for identifying possible solutions also uses a consistent framework. This framework consists of (1) identifying those people who should have input into the decision, (2) gathering all relevant facts and opinions from these people, (3) determining the available options, and finally, (4) selecting among the options using the patient's own values.

Legal and ethical issues and options have been defined and formulated from specific pivotal clinical cases. Widely publicized cases have focused the attention of the public, legal, and medical communities on major ethical questions. The cases of Karen Quinlan and Nancy Cruzan, for example, focused attention on the right to die and on who should ultimately make that decision. Concepts, such as informed consent, physician-assisted suicide, and health care rationing were not commonly discussed and in some cases were not even considered in the 1950s and 1960s. What has recently been called the "paternalistic autonomy" of the physician in the "golden age of medicine" to make unilateral medical decisions has evolved to the primacy of informed consent and shared decisionmaking.

A Short History of Ethical Thought

Beyond analyzing the nature of reality and the sources of knowledge, ethical philosophers deal with the concepts of right behavior, relationships between individuals, the nature of these relationships, and the priorities among these relationships. A number of philosophers have proposed theories that define the most common principles used in the practice of medical ethics.

The concepts of Immanuel Kant, a philosopher/moralist, are the basis of a substantial amount of ethical thought. Kant deduced a series of moral rules or maxims to define the nature of "right" action. He maintained that morality should be grounded in pure reason and should not be affected by conscience or sympathy; that is, decisions should be judged on their intentions and divorced of their consequences. Actions are to be judged as correct, regardless of the effect that they have on the real world or its inhabitants. These maxims were correct if they could be applied universally; that is, if they could apply to anyone in a similar situation.

Kant supported the concept of the intrinsic worth of human beings, thus supporting the concept of *autonomy* and *informed consent*, forbidding treatment or experimentation on a patient without his or her knowledge and expressed consent. According to Kant, good outcomes do not make an action morally right.

The British philosophers John Stuart Mill and Jeremy Bentham advanced the *theory of utilitarianism*. Essentially, the utility of actions "are right in proportion as they tend to promote happiness, wrong as they tend to produce the reverse of happiness." Unlike Kant's theory, the result of the action (increase in happiness) is the measurement against which an action is to be judged. No action can be judged categorically right or wrong; rather, it should be judged on the utility of the result: "Those actions are right that produce the greatest happiness for the greatest number of people."

More recent philosophers, including W. D. Ross, have attempted to incorporate aspects of Kant's and Mill's concepts. Ross believes his list of duties should be binding on all moral agents, including health care providers and administrators:

1. Truth telling
2. Reparation for wrongs
3. Justice (rewards or happiness based on merit)
4. Beneficence (improving the human condition by "doing good")
5. Nonmaleficence (avoiding or preventing harm or injury to others)

Circumstances in which these duties conflict with each other are easily imagined, however. Lying about a condition to an insurance company may get a patient necessary therapy to improve her health, but at the expense of truth telling. A sense of morality outside these duties helps with balancing the various concepts.

⬤ Ethical Principles in Medical Care

When considering ethical issues, many ethicists use the principles of beneficence, utility, nonmaleficence, and distributive justice. These principles have been derived from theories set forth by philosophers, including those discussed above. These concepts can be applied to ethical dilemmas to help see options, to determine priorities, and to make decisions.

The *principle of nonmaleficence* is related to acting in ways that do not result in needless harm or injury (avoiding harm or injury to others). Physicians know this as *primum non nocere* (first, do no harm). There is a corresponding legal requirement of avoiding negligence and providing the professional level of care expected of a practicing physician. Professionals are licensed and required to maintain their skills and keep current. Thus, practicing outside your area of expertise or training is unethical. Turning off a respirator at a family's request, without knowing the patient's wishes, would not be supportive of the patient's interests and could be harmful to the desires of the patient. Providing futile care that has no benefit but would cause pain or prolong the dying process might also be a harmful action.

To prevent doing harm, one must mentally perform a risk-benefit analysis before recommending a test or a course of action. The course may include costly tests that, although not painful, do not advance the diagnosis and serve only to enrich the physician, to decrease malpractice risk, or to involve the patient or insurance company without any benefit (with no utility of action). Reasonable choices must be taken so that the sum of the actions does not cause harm.

The *principle of beneficence* means that a physician should do more than just avoid harming the patient; he or she should actively help the patient. Such help is the essence of medical practice. Physicians have a commitment to help patients by taking the call, being available, helping them understand medical treatment, and promoting individual and public health goals. This principle could be considered to support and mandate caring for patients on public assistance, or charity cases in which the reimbursement is meager, if available at all. On a more universal level, this principle extends to the issues of providing care for the uninsured.

In a way, the *principle of utility* has its genesis from the previous two principles, in that actions should maximize benefit while minimizing harm. This principle mandates careful analysis of patient care and health care policy decisions to assure that the results serve both aims of utility. The most positive value or, if all options have negative ramifications, the least negative value, should guide decisionmaking. Maximizing the positive effects of providing health care, both preventive and "sick care," requires reviewing the way that funds are allocated as public policy, from the vantage point of society in general. What is the best allocation of health care dollars in a world of limited financial resources? In the case of Medicaid, do we expand the number of people covered and decrease the benefit package, or limit coverage and expand benefits? What benefit structure and eligibility criteria will result in maximizing the utility of this program for society?

The *principle of distributive justice* requires that we treat others justly and that we have a right to be treated justly in return. The unspoken caveat here is "all things being equal." The principle means that people should get that to which they are entitled. This principle could be construed to support physicians acting as patient advocates when a health plan rejects a proposed treatment (for pre-authorization) as being "not medically necessary." The corollary is also true; physicians should not falsify documentation to get patients services to which they are not entitled (services that are not a covered benefit) but that would help them medically. The moral philosophers support this principle as "truth telling," but it could be seen by some as conflicting with the principle of beneficence.

Distributive justice is also concerned with distribution of the health care dollar, the limited supply of ICU beds (i.e., who gets moved out to the floor), and how the limited supply of transplantable organs is allocated. Is health care a right or an economic service to which access is based on the ability to pay? Distributive justice maintains that similar cases should always be treated similarly. This sense of "fairness" argues against the early methods of allocating kidneys, in which some patients were judged "worthier" on the basis of socioeconomic status, societal value, or other attributes, rather than urgency or need. The thorniest issue is in determining when cases can be judged to be similar. How is this decision made—and which factors are to be considered and which are to be rejected? The principle of distributive justice can be used to determine whether certain policies are just, demonstrating that similar cases should be treated in a similar manner.

Another important ethical principle to consider is the *principle of equality*, supported by John Rawls, which maintains that benefits and burdens of society should be borne equally by all members of society. This principle could be seen as supporting a single-tier, universal health system into which all must participate with equal benefits and coverage, despite their ability to pay "more" for individualized (boutique) care.

A Three-Step Approach to Ethical Analysis

Analyzing ethical dilemmas in medicine requires both a framework and a method of analysis. Ethical principles and theories provide the framework; a three-step approach for analyzing ethical dilemmas is described below.

1. *Gather the facts of the case.* Clarify the facts, specific issues, situations, and differences of opinion of the case. Determine who are the appropriate decisionmakers and anyone else who should be involved in the process. This step should include learning the beliefs and opinions of the individuals involved and their understanding of the dilemma to be resolved. The involved parties need to explain why they believe or support particular actions or non-actions.

2. *Decide which ethical principles are the most relevant to the situation.* More than one principle can be considered, based on the specific circumstances of the case. For example, in analyzing the right of a patient to decline life-saving care or to terminate life-supporting care, one should do the following:

a) Review the patient's ability to exhibit autonomy; that is, determine whether he or she can make a decision. Has all pertinent information been provided in a form he or she can understand? Can he or she demonstrate an understanding of the information? Is the patient legally old enough to make the decision?

b) If the patient does not exhibit autonomy, is this inability to understand the result of a reversible condition, such as depression, bipolar disorder, psychosis, delirium, or other altered states caused by metabolic disease, medication, recreational drugs, or hypoxia? It is appropriate to treat the patient's medical or psychiatric condition, to determine if they can be improved to a point where they can comprehend the decision to be made and its impact on their clinical longevity, viability, and quality of life.

c) If the patient does not exhibit autonomy, is there an advance directive, health care proxy, living will, or other document recognized by the state in which the patient is hospitalized that expresses the patient's wishes before autonomy was lost?

d) If the patient does not exhibit autonomy, has he or she ever expressed an opinion concerning life-sustaining therapies? Would these opinions allow for a *substituted judgment*? (A substituted judgment requires the individual making this decision to "don the mental mantle" of the patient, attempting to determine what that individual would decide in the light of his or her value system, based on previously expressed wishes or opinions.) Using these values, he or she would determine what the individual would have decided if competent.

e) If no surrogate decisionmaker is available, determine whether the hospital should go to court to be awarded custody to make a decision. The court may make a decision based on substituted judgment or on the more generic concept of *best interest* (a less-specific judgment based not on what this patient would want but on what a "typical patient" in this situation would want). This position leaves the patient most open to the biases of the decisionmaker, who may be the hospital administrator or a judge. This position looks at the risks and benefits of this action to the patient. For example, is the therapy painful? Does it prolong dying without allowing the patient to experience happiness? Does it have a reasonable chance of benefiting the patient?

3. *Develop and present options based on the moral principles identified in # 2.* Once the facts and principles have been presented, the ethicist (as an impartial individual) can formulate the options, and those involved can decide which option to take.

Common Ethical Dilemmas

The most common ethical issues encountered by physicians include the need to:

1. provide informed consent for treatment
2. evaluate a patient's decision to decline medically necessary care
3. evaluate requests for futile or non-medically appropriate care
4. determine a patient's capacity for decisionmaking
5. come to terms with euthanasia or assisted suicide
6. respond to requests for termination of life-sustaining medication or therapies
7. decide on the distribution of scarce resources
8. engage in cost containment, resulting in restriction of care
9. understand confidentiality and privacy issues, including circumstances in which the patient's condition may put others at risk, such as when the patient is HIV-positive or expresses psychotic ideation
10. consider access to experimental or unproven therapy
11. care for terminally ill patients
12. care for infants, children, the mentally retarded, and people with dementia

Some of the issues mentioned above cannot be anticipated; however, many can be addressed with the patient before they become critical. As a physician or physician manager, it is important to obtain such documents as advance directives before the information is needed. A small amount of time invested on the front end of the patient-physician relationship can save much time and anguish for the patient, the family, administrators, and the physician.

Ethics Committees

Ethics consultants or ethics committees provide a number of different services for facilities by serving in a number of roles. These services include serving as a source of general education to hospital employees, acting as a convener of meetings to address ethical concerns of facility staff, serving as a consultant to physicians and other health care personnel on specifically problematic cases (where the right action is unclear to the physician in charge), reviewing actions or policies proposed by hospital staff, and advising patients and families concerning ethical and moral issues to facilitate communication with medical staff. Patients, in some cases, may not know a hospital ethics committee is discussing their cases. In general, physician ethicists function as ethicists first and clinicians second. Their role is not to oversee the patient's medical treatment.

An Ethical Dilemma Case: The Right to Die

Below is a short case history of a patient who presents an ethical dilemma to the hospital staff. Following the case history is an analysis of the ethical dilemmas and options of the case. This scenario is likely to become more frequent as the population ages. Who decides when care is futile, when "enough is enough"? Who chooses whether we live or die? Is it the patient, the caregivers, a court-appointed guardian, or the physician?

Case Study

Mary Elizabeth Wainwright, a lifetime smoker, has lived in a senior citizen high-rise for 27 years. At 93, she has outlived her husband and her son. She has no living relatives. She was brought to the ER by ambulance, short of breath but mentally alert. Her pulmonary condition has deteriorated, and she has been ventilator-dependent for the past two months. She is a favorite on the chronic vent unit, always smiling. The only problem for the staff is that she keeps pulling at her ET tube and repeatedly states that she wants the staff to let her die. Attempts to wean her from the ventilator have failed. Weekly, however, the staff attempts a "slow wean" off the ventilator.

The hospital is having difficulty finding a chronic vent unit to take her, as a result of her recently diagnosed brittle diabetes, severe rheumatoid arthritis, and ischemic cardiomyopathy. There are many opinions of what to do with her.

The intern on the case has stated to the nursing staff a number of times that "this is a futile case, why not shut off the ventilator? The money could be better spent elsewhere."

The hospital risk manager is concerned that if they honor her wishes and allow her to die, a relative may turn up who will "sue them." Therefore, he thinks it is better to continue the status quo.

The attending physician does not believe anyone would want to take his or her own life. "She must be delusional to want to die. I won't obey a crazy person's wishes."

The senior resident, who, with the intern, is the primary care team, is confused about what to do. She calls Dr. Jay, who is on the ethics committee and asks for his help.

The ethics committee meets, but before this meeting, a member of the committee meets with the patient. The patient communicates the following: "I have lived a long life and liked best to walk around, watering my plants and talking to my cat. All my friends and relatives have died. My eyesight and hearing are rapidly failing, and my joints hurt from being in bed so long." She stated that she expects more pain in the future, without significant improvement. She does not expect to be taken off the respirator or to walk around her apartment ever again. She has lived long enough and therefore chooses to die.

The ethics committee meets with the attending physician, resident, intern, and key nursing staff. The ethics committee member, who spoke with Mrs. Wainwright, provides the patient's rationale, and discusses the patient's wishes and her capacity to make a decision of this magnitude. The committee discusses concepts of nonmaleficence, beneficence, and her autonomy. Options are discussed as to what to do and how to best serve her interests.

This case touches on a number of ethical principles. If a treatment involves pain, repeated hospital visits, lab tests, or prolonged hospitalization, maximizing lifespan may be the physician's choice as he or she views maximizing happiness and beneficence for the patient; however, it may not have the same utility for an elderly patient. He or she may value overall freedom from pain and suffering or an escape from a prolonged final decline in a hospital or countless physician visits. The physician's quest to obtain tissue for the diagnosis of a terminal cancer, in which noxious treatments are likely to result in constant nausea and disfigurement, is likely not be valuable to an elderly patient. Compassion and the requirements of informed consent let patients make decisions based on their desires and personal values. Patient autonomy (i.e., doing no harm) based on the patient wishes should take priority.

Mrs. Wainwright was subsequently determined by a psychiatrist not to suffer from a psychiatric illness that would affect her decisionmaking capacity. She was informed about her condition and demonstrated a good understanding of her current situation. It was highly unlikely that she would be weaned from the ventilator and that she was severely limited in what she could do. She saw her life as ongoing suffering and derived no happiness from it. She made a rational decision based on her assessment of the situation and her values.

Physicians had nothing left to offer. She was rejecting what she and some of the staff saw as futile care. Even if she had had advance directives, a living will, or had assigned a health care power of attorney for someone else to make decisions if she was incapacitated, it would not apply in this case because she was capable of making her own decisions. Continuing her life was not providing her happiness or satisfaction and could be seen as harmful to her, causing psychic and physical harm. Providing medications to relieve pain would likely cause sedation and respiratory depression.

Treatment and prolongation of life in her current condition was not seen as being helpful or beneficial to her. These concepts were discussed with the staff. The medical care that the staff provided to prolong her life was actually seen as harmful. The house staff, attending physician, and representative nursing staff from the floor participated in the discussion and helped arrive at a decision.

The staff discussed the patient's choice of termination of life support with her one final time. She remained adamant. She was medicated with a low dose of morphine as needed for her unremitting arthritis pain and her weekly weaning began the next morning as scheduled. She would not be returned to the respirator. The next morning, the staff made sure she was kept comfortable during the weaning attempt and supported her request not to be placed back on the respirator.

Harm was prevented (nonmaleficence) by not continuing futile care that prolonged her suffering. It was the concept of beneficence that allowed the patient to exert autonomy in choosing life or death, after being informed realistically of her chances of a recovery and of returning to the activities that gave her happiness. Not returning the patient to the respirator had the highest utility for her.

References

1. Ariz. Admin. Code R9-22-204
2. 210 ILCS 85/10.4(b)
3. 42 C.F.R. § 482.21
4. 42 U.S.C. § 1395bb(a)
5. N.Y. Pub. Health Law § 4403(f)
6. 42 C.F.R. § 422.152(a)

7. 42 C.F.R. § 438.240(a)(1)

8. *Purcell v. Zimbelman*, 18 Ariz. App. 75, 500 P.2d 335 (1972)

9. *Blanton v. Moses H. Cone Memorial Hospital, Inc.*, 319 N.C. 372, 354 S.E.2d 455 (1987)

10. *Schlier v. Kaiser Found. Health Plan of the Mid-Atlantic States, Inc.*, 876 F.2d 174 (D.C. Cir. 1989)

11. *Boyd v. Albert Einstein Med. Ctr.*, 547 A.2d 1229 (Pa. Super. Ct. 1988); *Harell v. Total Care Healthcare, Inc.*, 781 S.W.2d 58 (Mo. 1989); *Petrovich v. Share Health Plan of Illinois, Inc.*, 696 N.E. 2d 356 (Ill. App. Ct. 1998)

12. *Villazon v. Prudential Health Care Plan, Inc.*, No. SC01-1397, 2003 WL 1561528 (Fla. Mar. 27, 2003)

13. 42 C.F.R. § 482.12(a)

14. A.R.S. § 36-445

15. 63 PA. Cons. Stat. Ann. § 425.4

16. A.R.S. § 36-2403

17. AMA H-375.989

18. *Humana Hospital Desert Valley v. Superior Court*, 154 Ariz. 396, 400, 742 P.2d 1382, 1386 (Ct. App. 1987) (citations omitted)

19. 63 PA. Cons. Stat. Ann. § 425.4

20. A.R.S. §§ 36-2401, 2402 and 2403

21. 63 PA. Cons. Stat. Ann. § 425.4

22. A.R.S. § 36-2403

23. 559 Pa. 21, 731 A.2d 114 (1999)

24. 259 F. 3d 284 (4th Cir 2001)

25. 2003 U.S. App. LEXIS 12719 (D.C. Cir. Jun. 20, 2003)

26. 42 U.S.C. § 1320c-3(a)(14)

27. Morter C, *The Health Care Quality Improvement Act of 1986: Will Physicians Find Peer Review More Inviting?*, 74 Va. L. Rev. 1115, 1115 (1988) (Discusses the reasons Congress passed the immunity provisions under the Health Care Quality Improvement Act of 1986, which is often referred to by its acronym, HCQIA.)

28. 42 U.S.C. § 11101

29. A.R.S. § 36-445.02(B)

30. 63 PA. Cons. Stat. Ann. § 425.3

31. 42 U.S.C. § 11111(a)(1)

32. 42 U.S.C. § 11112(a)

33. 42 U.S.C. § 11112(a)

34. *Bryan v. James E. Holmes Reg'l Med. Ctr.*, 33 F.3d 1318, 1333 (11th Cir. 1994)

35. *Matthews v. Lancaster General Hosp.*, 87 F.3d. 624, 628 (3d Cir. 1996)

36. *Meyers v. Columbia/HCA*, 341 F.3d 461 (6th Cir 2003)

37. *Brown v. Presbyterian Healthcare Services*, 101 F.3d 1324 (10th Cir.1996)

38. *Clark v. Columbia/HCA*, 25 P.3d 215 (Nev. 2001)

39. 42 U.S.C. § 11112(b)

40. 42 U.S.C. § 11112(a)(4); *Smith v. Ricks*, 31 F.3d 1478, 1486 (9th Cir.1994); and *Fobbs v. Holy Cross Health Sys. Corp.*, 29 F.3d 1439, 1445 (9th Cir.1994)

41. *Fact Sheet on the National Practitioner Data Bank* from the Health Resources & Services Administration of the U.S. Department of Health and Human Services Health Services, available at *www.npdb-hipdb.com*

42. 42 U.S.C. §§ 11131 through 11137

43. 45 C.F.R. § 60.3

44. 45 C.F.R. § 60.7

45. 45 C.F.R. § 60.8

46. 45 C.F.R. § 60.9

47. 45 C.F.R. § 60.9

● Suggested Readings

Ahronheim J, Moreno J, Zuckerman C. *Ethics in Clinical Practice*. Boston, MA: Little, Brown and Company; 1994.

Beauchamp T, Childress J. *Principles of Biomedical Ethics*. 4th ed. Oxford, England: Oxford University Press; 1994.

Fletcher J, Quist N, Jonsen A, eds. *Ethics Consultation in Health Care*. Ann Arbor, MI: Health Administration Press; 1989.

Morreim E. *Balancing Act: The New Medical Ethics of Medicine's New Economics*. Washington, DC: Georgetown University Press; 1995.

Munson R. *Interventions and Reflection: Basic Issues in Medical Ethics*. Belmont, CA: Wadsworth Publishing Company; 1992.

Schneider C. *The Practice of Autonomy: Patients, Doctors, and Medical Decisions*. Oxford, England: Oxford University Press; 1998.

Veach R. *A Theory of Medical Ethics*. New York, NY: Basic Books; 1981.

Wong K. *Medicine and the Marketplace: The Moral Dimensions of Managed Care*. South Bend, IN: University of Notre Dame Press; 1999.

INDEX